# Natural Pain Relief Without Opioids

## The Complete Guide to Alternative Pain Management

**Blanche Bryce Hoffman**

**ISBN: 978-1-7642100-1-0**

**Isohan Publishing**

# Table of Contents

# Chapter 1: The New Era of Natural Pain Relief

The medical establishment has reached a crossroads. After decades of relying on opioids as the primary solution for pain management, healthcare providers now face an undeniable truth: we need better answers. The statistics paint a sobering picture - more than 70,000 Americans died from drug overdoses in 2019 alone, with prescription opioids playing a significant role in this crisis (1). Yet simultaneously, millions of people continue to suffer from chronic pain, desperately seeking relief that doesn't come with the risk of addiction or death.

This shift represents more than just a change in prescribing habits. It signals a fundamental transformation in how we understand and treat pain itself. The old model - identify pain, prescribe medication, hope for the best - has given way to a more sophisticated approach that recognizes pain as a complex, multifaceted experience requiring equally complex solutions.

**Why This Book Matters Now**

The paradigm shift in pain management isn't happening in isolation. It's driven by mounting evidence that non-pharmacological approaches can be just as effective as traditional medications, often with fewer side effects and better long-term outcomes. The American College of Physicians now recommends non-drug therapies as first-line treatments for chronic low back pain (2). Similarly, the Centers for Disease Control and Prevention has updated its guidelines to emphasize non-opioid treatments for chronic pain (3).

This evidence-based revolution has created both opportunity and confusion. Patients find themselves overwhelmed by options - acupuncture, physical therapy, mindfulness meditation, dietary changes, and dozens of other approaches. Healthcare providers, trained in a system that emphasized pharmaceutical solutions, often lack the knowledge to guide patients through these alternatives effectively.

Consider Maria, a 45-year-old teacher who developed chronic neck pain after a car accident. Her initial treatment followed the traditional path: muscle relaxants, then stronger pain medications, eventually leading to opioid dependence. After three years of escalating medication use with diminishing returns, she found herself trapped in a cycle of increasing doses and increasing desperation. Her turning point came when she discovered a multimodal approach combining physical therapy, acupuncture, and cognitive behavioral therapy. Within six months, she had weaned off all pain medications and returned to work full-time.

**Meet Suzetrigine (Journavx)**

In January 2025, the FDA approved a medication that represents a genuine breakthrough in pain management. Suzetrigine, marketed as Journavx, works through an entirely different mechanism than opioids (4). Instead of binding to opioid receptors in the brain, it targets sodium channels in nerve cells, specifically the Nav1.8 channel that plays a crucial role in pain signaling.

This mechanism offers several advantages over traditional opioids. First, it doesn't carry the same risk of respiratory depression that makes opioid overdoses so dangerous. Second, it appears to have minimal potential for addiction or abuse. Third, clinical trials suggest it may be particularly effective for neuropathic pain conditions that often respond poorly to opioids (5).

The approval of suzetrigine validates a broader principle: effective pain relief doesn't require accepting the risks that come with opioid therapy. This medication represents just one example of how innovation in pain management is expanding beyond traditional pharmaceutical approaches.

Take David, a 62-year-old construction worker who developed severe neuropathic pain following a work-related injury. Traditional pain medications provided minimal relief while causing significant side effects including constipation, cognitive fog, and mood changes. When his physician prescribed suzetrigine as part of a broader pain management plan, David experienced substantial improvement in his pain levels without the troublesome side effects he'd experienced with opioids. The medication became one component of a comprehensive approach that also included physical therapy and workplace modifications.

## Your Roadmap to Relief

This book provides a systematic approach to pain management that goes beyond simply listing treatment options. Each chapter builds upon previous knowledge, creating a framework you can use to develop your own personalized pain management strategy.

The journey begins with understanding pain science - not because you need to become a neuroscientist, but because understanding how pain works helps you make informed decisions about treatment. From there, we explore physical approaches that can help restore function and reduce pain signals. Mind-body techniques follow, recognizing that pain exists at the intersection of physical sensation and psychological experience.

The book then addresses specific pain conditions, providing targeted strategies for common problems like back pain, arthritis, and headaches. Finally, we explore how to integrate these approaches into a comprehensive plan that fits your lifestyle and preferences.

Throughout this journey, you'll find practical tools and assessments to help you track your progress and adjust your approach as needed. The goal isn't to eliminate every sensation of discomfort - that's neither realistic nor necessarily desirable. Instead, we aim to reduce pain to manageable levels while improving your overall quality of life.

## Success Stories

Real-world examples demonstrate the effectiveness of comprehensive pain management approaches. These stories illustrate not just what's possible, but how ordinary people have transformed their relationship with pain using the principles outlined in this book.

Sarah, a 38-year-old mother of two, developed fibromyalgia after a series of stressful life events. Her initial treatment focused heavily on medication management, but side effects from the medications often felt worse than the pain itself. Working with a pain management team, she gradually implemented a multimodal approach including gentle exercise, stress management techniques, and dietary modifications. The process took time - nearly a year to see significant improvement - but the results were transformative. She now manages her condition with minimal medication while maintaining an active lifestyle.

Robert, a 55-year-old office worker, struggled with chronic low back pain for over a decade. Multiple surgeries had provided only temporary relief, and he faced the prospect of permanent disability. His breakthrough came through a combination of physical therapy focused on movement retraining, mindfulness-based stress reduction, and workplace ergonomic modifications. The key wasn't any single intervention, but rather the way these approaches worked together to address different aspects of his pain experience.

Jennifer, a 29-year-old nurse, developed complex regional pain syndrome following a minor hand injury. This condition often proves resistant to traditional treatments, and Jennifer's case was no exception. Her recovery involved a carefully coordinated approach including desensitization therapy, mirror therapy, and psychological support to address the fear and anxiety that had developed around her pain. The process required patience and persistence, but she eventually returned to work in a modified capacity and continues to improve.

**The Promise of Multimodal Treatment**

The success stories shared above illustrate a fundamental principle: comprehensive pain management works better than any single approach alone. This concept, known as multimodal treatment, recognizes that pain is a complex phenomenon requiring multiple interventions targeting different aspects of the pain experience.

Consider how pain affects your life. It's not just the physical sensation - it's the way pain disrupts sleep, affects mood, limits activities, and impacts relationships. A truly effective approach must address all these dimensions, not just the immediate sensation of discomfort.

Research consistently demonstrates that multimodal approaches produce better outcomes than single-modality treatments. A study published in the Journal of Pain found that patients receiving multimodal treatment for chronic pain showed greater improvements in pain intensity, functional ability, and quality of life compared to those receiving single treatments (6).

The key to successful multimodal treatment lies in understanding how different approaches complement each other. Physical therapy might address movement dysfunction and muscle imbalances. Cognitive behavioral therapy can help change unhelpful thought patterns that amplify pain. Mindfulness training develops skills for managing pain flares. Anti-inflammatory nutrition supports tissue healing. Each component contributes to the overall goal of reducing pain and improving function.

This approach also provides resilience. If one treatment stops working or becomes unavailable, you have other tools to rely on. This redundancy is particularly important for chronic pain conditions that may require long-term management.

The evidence supporting multimodal treatment continues to grow. The American Pain Society, before its dissolution, endorsed multimodal approaches as the standard of care for chronic pain management (7). Professional organizations across multiple disciplines now emphasize the importance of coordinated, comprehensive treatment plans.

**Building Your Foundation**

Starting this journey requires both hope and realism. The approaches outlined in this book have helped millions of people reduce their pain and improve their quality of life. However, finding the right combination of treatments for your specific situation takes time and patience.

Success in pain management often follows a pattern. Initial improvements may be modest, but they build upon each other over time. Small gains in sleep quality lead to better mood regulation. Improved mood makes it easier to engage in physical activity. Increased activity strengthens the body and builds confidence. This positive cycle can transform your relationship with pain.

The journey also requires active participation. Unlike taking a pill and waiting for relief, these approaches require your engagement and commitment. This isn't a burden - it's actually an advantage. By becoming an active participant in your own care, you develop skills and knowledge that serve you for life.

**Moving Forward**

The chapters that follow provide the tools and knowledge you need to create your own comprehensive pain management plan. Each section builds systematically, providing both theoretical understanding and practical applications.

You'll learn how pain signals travel through your nervous system and how you can influence these signals through various interventions. You'll discover evidence-based physical approaches that can restore function and reduce pain. You'll explore mind-body techniques that harness your brain's natural pain-fighting abilities.

Most importantly, you'll develop the confidence to take control of your pain rather than letting it control you. This shift from passive recipient to active participant represents one of the most powerful changes you can make in your relationship with pain.

The road ahead isn't always easy, but it's filled with possibility. Millions of people have found relief using the approaches outlined in this book. With patience, persistence, and the right tools, you can join them in creating a life where pain no longer defines your limits.

**Chapter Wrap-Up**

The transformation of pain management from a medication-focused approach to a comprehensive, multimodal strategy represents one of medicine's most significant advances. This shift acknowledges pain as a complex experience requiring equally sophisticated solutions. New medications like suzetrigine provide safer pharmaceutical options, while evidence-based non-drug approaches offer effective alternatives to traditional pain management.

Your journey toward better pain management starts with understanding that relief is possible without accepting the risks associated with long-term opioid use. The stories of Maria, David, Sarah, Robert, and Jennifer demonstrate that comprehensive approaches can produce lasting improvements in pain and quality of life.

**Key Takeaways:**

- Pain management has shifted from medication-only approaches to comprehensive, multimodal strategies

- New medications like suzetrigine offer effective pain relief without opioid-related risks

- Success in pain management requires active participation and patience with the process

- Multimodal treatment produces better outcomes than any single approach alone

- Evidence-based non-drug approaches can be as effective as traditional medications

- Real people have found lasting relief using the principles outlined in this book

# Chapter 2: Pain Science Made Simple

Understanding how pain works might seem like unnecessary complexity, but this knowledge becomes your most powerful tool for managing pain effectively. Most people think of pain as a simple alarm system - injury occurs, nerves send signals, brain receives message, person feels pain. The reality is far more sophisticated and, fortunately, far more hopeful.

Your pain experience depends not just on what's happening in your tissues, but on how your nervous system processes, interprets, and responds to signals. This processing can be influenced, modified, and even redirected through various interventions. Once you understand these mechanisms, you gain the ability to actively participate in your own pain relief.

**How Pain Actually Works**

The gate control theory, first proposed by Ronald Melzack and Patrick Wall in 1965, revolutionized our understanding of pain (8). This theory explains why rubbing an injury makes it feel better, why distraction can reduce pain, and why the same injury can feel different depending on your circumstances.

Imagine your spinal cord contains a gate that controls pain signals traveling to your brain. This gate can be opened or closed by various factors. When the gate is open, pain signals flow freely, and you experience more pain. When the gate is closed or partially closed, fewer pain signals reach your brain, and you feel less pain.

Several factors influence this gate. Non-painful sensations like touch, pressure, or vibration can close the gate - this explains why rubbing a bumped elbow provides relief. Distraction also closes the gate by occupying your brain's attention resources. Conversely, anxiety, depression, and focusing on pain can open the gate wider, increasing your pain experience.

Consider Tom, a 42-year-old accountant who developed chronic shoulder pain after a sports injury. Initially, his pain was manageable during busy workdays but became severe in the evenings when he had time to focus on it. This pattern illustrates gate control theory in action - his brain's engagement with work-related tasks partially closed the pain gate, while quiet evening hours allowed the gate to open wider.

The gate control theory also explains why pain can vary so dramatically between individuals with similar injuries. Two people with identical tissue damage may have completely different pain experiences based on how their nervous systems process the signals.

Modern neuroscience has expanded on this basic model, revealing that pain processing involves multiple brain regions working in concert. The anterior cingulate cortex processes the emotional aspects of pain, while the somatosensory cortex handles the sensory qualities like location and intensity. The prefrontal cortex contributes to pain's cognitive aspects, including attention and meaning-making (9).

This distributed processing explains why pain feels different in different contexts. A paper cut during an important presentation barely registers, while the same cut might throb painfully during a quiet moment at home. The physical stimulus is identical, but the brain's processing changes based on context, attention, and competing demands.

**Acute vs. Chronic Pain**

Understanding the distinction between acute and chronic pain is crucial for effective pain management. These aren't just different durations of the same phenomenon - they represent fundamentally different biological processes requiring different treatment approaches.

Acute pain serves a protective function. It alerts you to injury, motivates you to seek help, and encourages behaviors that promote healing. This type of pain typically correlates well with tissue damage and decreases as healing progresses. Acute pain responds predictably to standard treatments like rest, ice, and anti-inflammatory medications.

Chronic pain, defined as pain lasting longer than three months, represents a different beast entirely. The original injury may have healed completely, but the pain persists due to changes in the nervous system itself. In chronic pain, the alarm system becomes hypersensitive, sending danger signals even when no threat exists.

Lisa, a 35-year-old teacher, illustrates this distinction clearly. She initially developed back pain after lifting heavy boxes during a classroom move. For the first few weeks, her pain followed a predictable pattern - worse with movement, better with rest, gradually improving as her strained muscles healed. However, after two months, her pain began following different rules. Some days she felt fine, others she could barely move, with no clear relationship to her activities. Her acute injury had resolved, but chronic pain mechanisms had taken over.

The transition from acute to chronic pain involves several neurological changes. Initially, pain signals travel along well-defined pathways. Over time, these pathways become more sensitive, requiring less stimulation to produce pain signals. New neural connections form, expanding the pain network and making it easier to activate. This process, called central sensitization, transforms the nervous system from a reliable alarm system into a hypersensitive detector that reports danger even when none exists.

Research shows that preventing this transition requires early, aggressive intervention. The first three months after injury represent a critical window during which appropriate treatment can prevent the development of chronic pain. This explains why modern pain management emphasizes early mobilization, stress reduction, and return to normal activities rather than extended rest periods.

**Central Sensitization Explained**

Central sensitization represents one of the most important concepts in modern pain science. This process transforms your normally protective pain system into a source of ongoing suffering. Understanding central sensitization helps explain why chronic pain often seems disproportionate to apparent tissue damage and why traditional treatments sometimes fail.

In a normal nervous system, pain signals must reach a certain threshold before they're transmitted to the brain. Central sensitization lowers this threshold, allowing weak signals that would normally be ignored to trigger pain responses. Simultaneously, it amplifies signals that do reach the brain, making them feel more intense than they should.

This process involves multiple changes throughout the nervous system. In the spinal cord, nerve cells become more excitable and develop new connections. In the brain, regions responsible for pain processing become hyperactive and expand their territory. The result is a pain system stuck in overdrive, constantly scanning for threats and interpreting normal sensations as dangerous.

Mark, a 48-year-old construction worker, experienced central sensitization after a workplace injury. Initially, his pain was limited to his injured back. Over months, however, he began experiencing pain in areas that hadn't been injured. Light touch became uncomfortable, and activities that should have been painless now caused significant discomfort. His nervous system had become hypersensitive, misinterpreting normal sensations as threats.

Central sensitization also explains why pain can spread beyond the original injury site. The hypersensitive nervous system begins interpreting signals from surrounding areas as painful. This phenomenon, called secondary hyperalgesia, can make it seem like the original problem is getting worse when it's actually the pain processing system that has changed.

The good news is that central sensitization can be reversed. Just as the nervous system learned to become hypersensitive, it can learn to return to normal sensitivity. This process, called desensitization, forms the foundation of many successful chronic pain treatments.

Desensitization typically involves gradually exposing the nervous system to previously painful stimuli in a controlled, safe manner. Physical therapy uses graded exposure to movement. Cognitive behavioral therapy addresses fearful thoughts that maintain hypersensitivity. Mindfulness training helps distinguish between actual threats and false alarms from an overactive pain system.

**The Mind-Body Connection**

The connection between psychological factors and pain experience isn't just theoretical - it's measurable and clinically significant. Brain imaging studies show that thoughts, emotions, and expectations directly influence pain processing regions in the brain. This connection works both ways: pain affects mood and thinking, while mood and thinking affect pain intensity.

Stress hormones like cortisol and adrenaline can sensitize pain pathways, making you more susceptible to pain. Chronic stress keeps these hormones elevated, creating a biological environment that promotes pain persistence. Conversely, relaxation techniques that reduce stress hormone levels can decrease pain sensitivity.

Depression and anxiety don't just coexist with chronic pain - they actively worsen it. These conditions alter brain chemistry in ways that amplify pain signals and impair the brain's natural pain-fighting mechanisms. Treating depression and anxiety often produces substantial improvements in pain levels, even when the underlying injury hasn't changed.

Consider Jennifer, a 44-year-old nurse who developed chronic headaches during a particularly stressful period at work. Her headaches seemed to follow no pattern - they occurred regardless of her sleep, diet, or physical activity. However, they consistently worsened during high-stress periods and improved during vacations. Her pain was real and physical, but its triggers were primarily psychological.

The placebo effect demonstrates the mind-body connection in its most dramatic form. Patients receiving inactive treatments often experience genuine pain relief, sometimes comparable to active medications. This isn't "just in their heads" - brain scans show that placebo treatments activate the same pain-relieving pathways as actual medications.

Understanding this connection empowers you to use your mind as a tool for pain management. Techniques like meditation, guided imagery, and cognitive restructuring can produce measurable changes in pain intensity and brain activity. These approaches work not by changing your thoughts about pain, but by changing how your brain processes pain signals.

**Neuroplasticity: Your Brain's Superpower for Healing**

Neuroplasticity - the brain's ability to reorganize and form new neural connections - represents perhaps the most hopeful aspect of pain science. This discovery has revolutionized treatment approaches and offers genuine hope for people with chronic pain conditions.

For decades, scientists believed that adult brains were fixed and unchangeable. We now know this is false. Your brain constantly rewires itself based on experience, thoughts, and activities. This process continues throughout life, meaning that negative changes associated with chronic pain can be reversed.

Chronic pain literally changes brain structure. Areas responsible for pain processing become larger and more active, while regions involved in mood regulation and executive function shrink. However, these changes aren't permanent. Appropriate interventions can restore normal brain structure and function (10).

Physical activity promotes neuroplasticity by stimulating the production of brain-derived neurotrophic factor (BDNF), a protein that supports nerve growth and repair. Exercise also increases production of endorphins, the body's natural pain-relieving chemicals. These effects explain why physical therapy remains one of the most effective treatments for chronic pain.

Mental training produces similar neuroplastic changes. Meditation increases gray matter density in areas associated with pain regulation while decreasing activity in pain-processing regions. Cognitive behavioral therapy helps rewire thought patterns that maintain chronic pain. Even learning new skills can promote positive brain changes that reduce pain sensitivity.

Susan, a 52-year-old office manager, utilized neuroplasticity principles in her recovery from chronic neck pain. Her treatment program included physical therapy to retrain movement patterns, meditation to promote relaxation responses, and cognitive therapy to address fear-based thinking. Brain scans taken before and after treatment showed measurable changes in pain-processing regions, corresponding to her significant improvement in symptoms.

The time required for neuroplastic changes varies, but research suggests that consistent practice for 8-12 weeks can produce lasting brain changes. This timeline helps explain why successful pain management requires patience and persistence - you're literally rewiring your brain, which takes time.

**Putting It All Together**

These pain science concepts work together to create a comprehensive understanding of your pain experience. The gate control theory explains why certain interventions provide immediate relief. The distinction between acute and chronic pain helps you understand why different approaches are needed for different situations. Central sensitization explains why chronic pain often seems disproportionate to apparent damage. The mind-body connection shows how psychological factors influence pain intensity. Neuroplasticity provides hope that negative changes can be reversed.

This knowledge transforms you from a passive recipient of pain to an active participant in your recovery. You understand that pain doesn't always correlate with tissue damage, that your nervous system can be retrained, and that your thoughts and emotions directly influence your pain experience.

Armed with this understanding, you can make informed decisions about treatment options. You know that addressing only the physical aspects of pain may not be sufficient for chronic conditions. You understand that treatments targeting the nervous system, emotions, and thought patterns aren't addressing "imaginary" pain - they're addressing the real biological processes that maintain chronic pain.

## Looking Ahead

The scientific understanding of pain continues to evolve rapidly. New discoveries about pain processing, neural plasticity, and the connections between mind and body are constantly expanding treatment possibilities. What remains constant is the central role of the nervous system in pain experience and the potential for positive change through appropriate interventions.

The next chapter will explore how these pain science principles translate into real-world impacts, examining the scope of chronic pain in America and the societal costs of inadequate treatment. Understanding these broader implications helps contextualize your personal pain experience within the larger healthcare landscape.

## Key Takeaways:

- Pain is processed by your nervous system, not just your tissues, making it modifiable through various interventions

- The gate control theory explains why distraction, touch, and other factors can reduce pain intensity

- Chronic pain involves changes in the nervous system itself, requiring different treatment approaches than acute pain

- Central sensitization makes your pain system hypersensitive, but this process can be reversed

- Your thoughts, emotions, and stress levels directly influence pain intensity through measurable brain changes

- Neuroplasticity means your brain can reorganize and heal throughout life, offering hope for recovery

# Chapter 3: The Truth About Chronic Pain in America

The numbers tell a story that healthcare providers and policymakers can no longer ignore. Chronic pain affects more Americans than diabetes, heart disease, and cancer combined, yet it receives a fraction of the attention and resources dedicated to these conditions. This disparity has created a silent epidemic that touches every corner of American society, from individual families struggling with medical bills to employers dealing with productivity losses to healthcare systems overwhelmed by complex cases.

Understanding the scope and impact of chronic pain in America isn't just academic exercise - it's essential for recognizing that your pain experience is part of a larger pattern that affects millions of people. This recognition can reduce the isolation and self-blame that often accompany chronic pain while highlighting the urgent need for better solutions.

**By the Numbers**

The latest data from the Centers for Disease Control and Prevention reveals the staggering scope of chronic pain in America. According to the 2023 National Health Interview Survey, approximately 58.5 million American adults experienced chronic pain in the past year, with 25.3 million experiencing high-impact chronic pain that significantly limits daily activities (11). These numbers represent substantial increases from previous years, suggesting that the problem is growing rather than improving.

To put these figures in perspective, chronic pain affects roughly one in five American adults. This prevalence exceeds that of diabetes (11.3%), heart disease (6.2%), and cancer (5.6%) combined. Yet chronic pain receives substantially less research funding and public attention than these other conditions.

The distribution of chronic pain isn't uniform across populations. Women experience chronic pain more frequently than men, with rates of 21.7% versus 19.0% respectively. Age also plays a significant role, with chronic pain affecting 10.6% of adults aged 18-29 but rising to 30.8% among those 65 and older. These demographic patterns reflect both biological differences and the cumulative effects of injuries and degenerative conditions over time.

Geographic variations reveal additional disparities. Rural areas report higher rates of chronic pain than urban centers, likely reflecting differences in occupational hazards, access to healthcare, and socioeconomic factors. The South and Midwest show particularly high rates, while the Northeast and West Coast tend to have lower prevalence.

Educational attainment strongly correlates with chronic pain rates. Adults with less than a high school education report chronic pain at rates nearly double those with college degrees. This relationship reflects the complex interplay between socioeconomic status, occupational exposures, and health outcomes.

Consider the case of Robert, a 58-year-old factory worker from rural Ohio. His chronic back pain developed gradually over decades of heavy lifting and repetitive motions. Limited healthcare access in his area meant delayed treatment, allowing acute injuries to progress to chronic conditions. His story illustrates how geographic, economic, and occupational factors combine to create higher chronic pain rates in certain populations.

The economic implications extend far beyond individual medical expenses. Chronic pain costs the American economy an estimated $635 billion annually in direct medical expenses and lost productivity (12). This figure exceeds the annual costs of cancer, heart disease, and diabetes combined, making chronic pain one of the most expensive health conditions in the United States.

**The Hidden Costs**

While the direct medical costs of chronic pain are substantial, the indirect costs often exceed them. Lost productivity represents the largest component of chronic pain's economic impact, accounting for approximately 61% of total costs. This includes not just missed workdays, but also reduced productivity while at work, a phenomenon known as presenteeism.

The workplace impact extends beyond individual suffering. Employers face increased healthcare premiums, higher absenteeism rates, and reduced productivity from affected employees. Small businesses, which often lack comprehensive health benefits, may struggle to retain skilled workers who develop chronic pain conditions.

Healthcare utilization patterns reveal the complexity of treating chronic pain. Patients with chronic pain visit healthcare providers twice as often as those without pain, and they're more likely to require emergency department care. These patterns strain healthcare systems already operating at capacity while often failing to provide effective relief for patients.

The prescription opioid crisis emerged partly from well-intentioned efforts to address undertreated pain. In the 1990s, medical organizations began emphasizing pain as the "fifth vital sign," encouraging more aggressive treatment of pain complaints. This approach, combined with misleading information about opioid addiction risks, led to dramatic increases in opioid prescribing.

The consequences have been devastating. From 1999 to 2019, more than 247,000 Americans died from prescription opioid overdoses (13). The crisis has since evolved to include heroin and synthetic opioids like fentanyl, but prescription opioids remain a significant factor in ongoing overdose deaths.

Sarah, a 34-year-old teacher, experienced this trajectory firsthand. Her chronic pain began with a back injury that was initially treated with short-term opioid therapy. As her pain persisted, her prescriptions increased in strength and duration. Within two years, she found herself dependent on opioids while experiencing minimal pain relief. Her recovery required medical detoxification, addiction treatment, and a complete restructuring of her pain management approach.

The opioid crisis has created a pendulum effect in pain treatment. Many healthcare providers, fearful of contributing to addiction problems, have become reluctant to prescribe any pain medications. This approach has left many patients with legitimate pain conditions undertreated, creating a different but equally serious problem.

**Dispelling Common Myths**

Misconceptions about chronic pain persist in both medical and public consciousness, creating barriers to effective treatment and social support. These myths often stem from outdated understanding of pain mechanisms and can significantly impact how people with chronic pain are perceived and treated.

**Myth 1: Pain always indicates tissue damage.** This belief, while true for acute pain, doesn't apply to chronic pain conditions. Many people with chronic pain have no detectable tissue damage, while others with significant structural abnormalities experience no pain. Brain imaging studies consistently show that chronic pain involves changes in pain processing systems rather than ongoing tissue damage.

**Myth 2: Chronic pain is "just in your head."** This harmful misconception suggests that chronic pain is imaginary or exaggerated. In reality, chronic pain involves measurable changes in brain structure and function. The pain is real and physical, even when psychological factors contribute to its maintenance.

**Myth 3: Rest is the best treatment for chronic pain.** While rest is appropriate for acute injuries, prolonged inactivity often worsens chronic pain. Extended rest leads to muscle deconditioning, joint stiffness, and increased pain sensitivity. Modern pain management emphasizes gradual return to activity rather than prolonged rest.

**Myth 4: Stronger pain medications are always better.** The relationship between medication strength and pain relief isn't linear. Higher doses often produce diminishing returns while increasing side effects and addiction risks. Effective pain management focuses on optimizing function rather than eliminating all pain sensations.

**Myth 5: Chronic pain is a normal part of aging.** While pain becomes more common with age, it's not an inevitable consequence of getting older. Many age-related pain conditions can be effectively treated or prevented through appropriate interventions.

Michael, a 67-year-old retiree, initially accepted his chronic knee pain as an inevitable part of aging. This belief prevented him from seeking treatment for months, allowing his condition to worsen. Once he learned that his pain was treatable, he pursued physical therapy and lost weight, resulting in significant improvement in his symptoms.

These myths create real harm by delaying appropriate treatment, increasing stigma, and reducing social support for people with chronic pain. Healthcare providers may dismiss patients' complaints, family members may question the reality of invisible pain, and employers may question the legitimacy of work limitations.

**The Opioid Crisis Context**

The opioid crisis has fundamentally altered the landscape of pain management in America. Understanding this context is crucial for anyone dealing with chronic pain, as it affects everything from prescribing practices to insurance coverage to public perception of pain treatment.

The crisis began in the 1990s when pharmaceutical companies aggressively marketed opioid medications as safe and effective for chronic pain. Medical organizations, concerned about undertreated pain, endorsed more liberal use of these medications. The result was a dramatic increase in opioid prescribing, with prescription rates quadrupling between 1999 and 2010.

Initially, this increased prescribing was seen as progress in pain management. Patients who had previously suffered in silence finally had access to effective pain relief. However, it soon became clear that opioids carried significant risks that had been downplayed or ignored.

The transition from prescription opioids to illicit drugs represents one of the crisis's most tragic aspects. Many people who became dependent on prescription opioids eventually turned to heroin or fentanyl when their prescriptions were discontinued or became too expensive. This progression has contributed to the current overdose epidemic, which kills more than 80,000 Americans annually.

The healthcare system's response has been mixed. New prescribing guidelines emphasize caution and limit opioid prescriptions, but they often fail to provide adequate alternatives. Many patients who were stable on opioid therapy have had their medications reduced or eliminated without access to effective alternatives.

Dr. Jennifer Martinez, a pain management specialist, describes the challenging balance she faces daily: "I see patients who genuinely need pain relief, but I also see the devastating effects of opioid addiction. We need better options that provide effective pain control without the risks associated with opioids."

The regulatory response has included prescription monitoring programs, abuse-deterrent formulations, and increased oversight of prescribing practices. While these measures have reduced inappropriate prescribing, they've also created barriers for patients with legitimate pain conditions.

**Hope Through Innovation**

Despite the challenges facing pain management, significant innovations offer hope for better treatments. Research into pain mechanisms has accelerated dramatically, leading to new understanding of how chronic pain develops and persists.

The approval of suzetrigine represents just one example of how pharmaceutical innovation is expanding beyond traditional opioid approaches. This medication targets specific sodium channels involved in pain signaling, offering effective relief without the risks associated with opioid therapy.

Non-pharmaceutical innovations are equally promising. Virtual reality therapy has shown remarkable effectiveness for various pain conditions, working by redirecting attention and promoting relaxation. Wearable devices can now provide transcutaneous electrical nerve stimulation (TENS) therapy throughout the day, offering continuous pain relief.

Telemedicine has expanded access to specialized pain care, particularly important for rural populations. Patients can now consult with pain specialists, receive cognitive behavioral therapy, and participate in exercise programs from their homes. This technology became particularly valuable during the COVID-19 pandemic and continues to expand access to care.

Precision medicine approaches are beginning to personalize pain treatment. Genetic testing can identify individuals who metabolize certain medications differently, allowing for more targeted prescribing. Brain imaging techniques may eventually allow providers to predict which treatments will be most effective for individual patients.

The integration of artificial intelligence in pain management shows promise for improving diagnosis and treatment selection. Machine learning algorithms can analyze complex patterns in patient data to identify optimal treatment approaches. These tools may help providers navigate the complexity of chronic pain more effectively.

Lisa, a 29-year-old software developer, benefited from several of these innovations. Her chronic migraines were treated with a combination of a new CGRP inhibitor medication, virtual reality therapy for stress management, and a smartphone app that helped her track triggers and symptoms. This integrated approach, unavailable just a few years ago, allowed her to return to work full-time.

Research into the social determinants of pain is revealing how factors like housing quality, food security, and social support affect pain outcomes. This understanding is leading to more comprehensive approaches that address these underlying factors alongside medical treatment.

**The Path Forward**

The current state of chronic pain in America presents both challenges and opportunities. The scope of the problem is vast, but increased awareness is driving innovation and investment in solutions. The opioid crisis, while tragic, has focused attention on the need for better pain management approaches.

Success in addressing chronic pain will require coordinated efforts across multiple sectors. Healthcare providers need better training in pain management and access to evidence-based treatments. Researchers must continue developing new therapeutic approaches. Policymakers need to ensure that regulations support appropriate pain treatment while preventing abuse.

Patients and advocates play crucial roles in this transformation. By sharing their experiences and demanding better care, they can drive changes in how pain is understood and treated. Support groups and patient organizations provide platforms for advocacy and mutual support.

The workplace represents another important arena for change. Employers who invest in ergonomic improvements, stress reduction programs, and comprehensive health benefits can prevent many pain conditions from developing. Those who provide accommodation and support for employees with chronic pain conditions can reduce disability rates and improve outcomes.

Education remains fundamental to progress. Healthcare providers need better training in pain science and evidence-based treatments. Patients need access to accurate information about their conditions and treatment options. The general public needs better understanding of chronic pain to reduce stigma and increase support for affected individuals.

## Moving Forward Together

The statistics and trends outlined in this chapter paint a picture of a healthcare system struggling to address one of the most common and costly health conditions in America. Yet within this challenge lies opportunity - the chance to create a more effective, compassionate, and sustainable approach to pain management.

Your experience with chronic pain connects you to millions of others facing similar challenges. This shared experience can provide comfort and motivation while highlighting the urgent need for better solutions. By understanding the broader context of chronic pain in America, you can better advocate for yourself and others while working toward a future where effective pain management is accessible to all who need it.

**Pathways to Progress**

The transformation of pain management in America requires recognition that current approaches aren't meeting the needs of the millions of people living with chronic pain. This recognition is driving innovation in treatment approaches, research methodologies, and healthcare delivery systems.

The next chapter will explore how this scientific understanding translates into practical movement-based interventions. Physical approaches to pain management offer some of the most effective and safest treatments available, with evidence supporting their use across a wide range of pain conditions.

**Key Takeaways:**

- Chronic pain affects 58.5 million American adults, exceeding the prevalence of diabetes, heart disease, and cancer combined

- The economic impact of chronic pain reaches $635 billion annually in direct costs and lost productivity

- Common myths about chronic pain create barriers to effective treatment and social support

- The opioid crisis has complicated pain management but has also driven innovation in safer alternatives

- Demographic disparities in pain prevalence reflect complex interactions between social, economic, and occupational factors

- Innovation in pain management offers hope for more effective, safer treatment approaches

# Chapter 4: Movement as Medicine

Your body was designed to move. This isn't some philosophical statement - it's a biological fact supported by decades of research. The human musculoskeletal system evolved over millions of years to support complex movement patterns, and modern sedentary lifestyles have disrupted these natural patterns in ways that directly contribute to pain and dysfunction.

The evidence supporting movement-based interventions for pain management is overwhelming. Studies consistently demonstrate that appropriate physical activity can be more effective than medications for many chronic pain conditions. Yet many people with pain instinctively avoid movement, fearing it will worsen their condition. This protective response, while understandable, often perpetuates the very problem it seeks to avoid.

**Physical Therapy Fundamentals**

Physical therapy represents the cornerstone of evidence-based pain management. Unlike passive treatments that do something to you, physical therapy teaches you to actively participate in your recovery. This distinction is crucial because it builds skills and knowledge that serve you long after formal treatment ends.

The fundamental principle underlying physical therapy is that movement dysfunction contributes to pain, and correcting these dysfunctions can reduce pain while improving function. This approach addresses the root causes of pain rather than just managing symptoms.

Modern physical therapy has evolved far beyond simple exercises and stretches. Today's evidence-based practice incorporates pain science education, manual therapy techniques, movement analysis, and psychosocial support. This comprehensive approach recognizes that pain is a complex experience requiring multifaceted intervention.

Research supports physical therapy's effectiveness across numerous pain conditions. A systematic review published in the Journal of International Crisis and Risk Communication Research found that physical therapy interventions significantly reduced pain intensity and improved functional outcomes in patients with chronic pain conditions (14). The benefits extended beyond the treatment period, with many patients maintaining improvements six months or more after completing therapy.

**Case Example: Margaret's Transformation**

Margaret, a 52-year-old office manager, developed chronic neck and shoulder pain after years of poor posture and repetitive computer work. Her pain had gradually worsened over two years, reaching the point where she couldn't turn her head without significant discomfort. Sleep became difficult, and she found herself taking increasing amounts of over-the-counter pain medications.

Her physical therapist began with a comprehensive assessment that revealed multiple contributing factors: forward head posture, rounded shoulders, weak deep neck flexors, and tight chest muscles. More importantly, Margaret had developed fear-avoidance behaviors - she moved carefully and avoided activities that might trigger pain.

Treatment began with education about pain mechanisms and the role of movement in recovery. Margaret learned that her pain didn't necessarily indicate tissue damage and that appropriate movement could actually reduce her pain levels. This understanding was crucial for her willingness to participate in treatment.

The physical therapy program addressed multiple components simultaneously. Manual therapy techniques helped restore normal joint mobility and reduce muscle tension. Specific exercises targeted weakened muscles while stretching tight structures. Postural training taught Margaret how to position herself during computer work to prevent symptom recurrence.

Perhaps most importantly, the program included graded exposure to previously avoided activities. Margaret gradually returned to activities she had stopped due to pain, building confidence while demonstrating that movement was safe and beneficial.

After eight weeks of treatment, Margaret reported a 70% reduction in pain intensity and had returned to all her previous activities. Six months later, she maintained these improvements while continuing her home exercise program. Her case illustrates how physical therapy can break the cycle of pain and dysfunction that characterizes many chronic conditions.

## The Science Behind Movement Therapy

Movement therapy works through multiple mechanisms that address different aspects of the pain experience. Understanding these mechanisms helps explain why physical therapy can be so effective for pain management.

At the tissue level, appropriate movement promotes healing by increasing blood flow, reducing inflammation, and stimulating the production of healing factors. Movement also helps maintain tissue health by preventing the formation of adhesions and maintaining normal tissue elasticity.

The nervous system responds to movement in ways that directly affect pain processing. Physical activity stimulates the production of endorphins, the body's natural pain-relieving chemicals. Movement also activates descending pain inhibitory pathways that reduce pain signal transmission to the brain.

Movement therapy addresses the psychological aspects of pain through several mechanisms. Successful completion of movement tasks builds self-efficacy and confidence. The rhythmic nature of many exercises can induce relaxation responses that reduce anxiety and stress. Group exercise settings provide social support and normalization of the pain experience.

## Exercise Protocols That Work

Not all exercise is created equal for pain management. The type, intensity, and progression of exercise must be carefully tailored to individual needs and capabilities. Generic exercise prescriptions often fail because they don't account for the specific impairments and limitations associated with different pain conditions.

## Aerobic Exercise for Pain Relief

Aerobic exercise represents one of the most effective interventions for chronic pain. Research demonstrates that regular aerobic activity can reduce pain intensity, improve mood, and enhance quality of life across multiple pain conditions. The optimal prescription typically involves moderate-intensity exercise performed for 30-45 minutes, three to five times per week.

The key to successful aerobic exercise for pain management lies in proper progression. Many people with chronic pain have become deconditioned, making it crucial to start at appropriate intensity levels and progress gradually. The "start low, go slow" approach prevents symptom flares while building tolerance for increased activity.

## Case Example: Robert's Running Revival

Robert, a 45-year-old accountant, had been an avid runner until chronic low back pain forced him to stop all physical activity. Over two years, his pain worsened while his fitness declined dramatically. He gained weight, developed depression, and found himself caught in a cycle of pain and inactivity.

His physical therapist recommended a gradual return to aerobic exercise, starting with five-minute walks on a treadmill. Robert initially resisted, convinced that any activity would worsen his pain. However, he agreed to try the program after learning about the pain-relieving effects of aerobic exercise.

The progression was carefully structured. Robert began with five-minute walks at a comfortable pace, gradually increasing duration by two minutes each week. After four weeks, he was walking for 15 minutes without increased pain. At six weeks, he added brief jogging intervals.

The breakthrough came at week eight when Robert realized his pain levels were lower on exercise days than on rest days. This discovery motivated him to continue progressing, and within three months, he was running continuously for 30 minutes. His pain had decreased by 60%, and he had lost 20 pounds.

Robert's case demonstrates several important principles. First, the progression was gradual enough to avoid symptom flares. Second, the activity was enjoyable and meaningful to him, promoting long-term adherence. Third, he experienced direct feedback about exercise benefits, which motivated continued participation.

## Strength Training for Pain Management

Strength training offers unique benefits for pain management by addressing specific muscle imbalances and movement dysfunctions. Research shows that targeted strengthening exercises can reduce pain intensity while improving functional capacity in people with chronic pain conditions.

The approach to strength training for pain management differs significantly from traditional fitness training. The focus is on correcting specific impairments rather than maximizing strength gains. Exercises are selected based on individual assessment findings and progressed according to symptom response.

## Movement Pattern Training

Many pain conditions result from faulty movement patterns rather than specific structural problems. Movement pattern training teaches people to move in ways that reduce stress on painful structures while promoting optimal function.

This approach involves breaking down complex movements into component parts, correcting dysfunctional patterns, and then integrating the corrected movements into functional activities. The process requires careful attention to detail and consistent practice to establish new motor patterns.

## Yoga and Tai Chi for Pain Relief

Ancient movement practices like yoga and tai chi have gained recognition as effective treatments for chronic pain. These practices combine physical movement with mental focus and breathing techniques, creating a comprehensive approach to pain management.

The National Center for Complementary and Integrative Health has reviewed extensive research on yoga for pain management, concluding that yoga can be helpful for chronic low back pain, neck pain, and arthritis (15). UCLA Health has similarly endorsed these practices as evidence-based treatments for various pain conditions (16).

**Case Example: Linda's Yoga Journey**

Linda, a 58-year-old teacher, developed fibromyalgia following a stressful divorce. Her pain was widespread and unpredictable, making it difficult to maintain regular exercise routines. Traditional exercises often triggered symptom flares, leading to a pattern of starting and stopping various activities.

Her physician recommended yoga as a gentler alternative that might be better tolerated. Linda was initially skeptical, viewing yoga as too "new age" for her practical nature. However, she agreed to try a therapeutic yoga class designed specifically for people with chronic pain.

The class began with basic breathing exercises and gentle stretches. The instructor emphasized listening to the body and modifying poses as needed. Linda appreciated this approach, which differed dramatically from her previous exercise experiences that focused on pushing through discomfort.

Over several weeks, Linda noticed gradual improvements in her flexibility and pain levels. More importantly, she began to sleep better and felt less anxious about her condition. The mindfulness component of yoga helped her develop a different relationship with her pain, viewing it as information rather than a threat.

After six months of regular yoga practice, Linda reported significant improvements in pain intensity, sleep quality, and mood. She had also developed a community of support through her yoga class, connecting with others who understood her experience. Her case illustrates how yoga's combination of physical movement and mental training can address multiple aspects of chronic pain.

## The Mechanisms of Mind-Body Movement

Yoga and tai chi work through multiple mechanisms that address both physical and psychological aspects of pain. The slow, controlled movements help improve flexibility, strength, and balance while promoting relaxation and stress reduction.

The breathing techniques taught in these practices activate the parasympathetic nervous system, promoting relaxation and reducing stress hormones that can amplify pain. The mindfulness component helps people develop better awareness of their bodies and pain patterns, leading to more effective self-management.

Research has identified specific neurological changes associated with yoga and tai chi practice. Brain imaging studies show increased activity in regions associated with pain regulation and decreased activity in areas associated with pain processing. These changes correspond to reported improvements in pain intensity and quality of life.

## Pilates for Pain Management

Pilates offers a unique approach to pain management by focusing on core stability, postural alignment, and movement quality. Originally developed as a rehabilitation method, Pilates has evolved into an evidence-based treatment for various pain conditions.

The Pilates method emphasizes controlled, precise movements that target deep stabilizing muscles often neglected in traditional exercise programs. This focus on core stability is particularly relevant for spinal pain conditions, where instability and poor motor control contribute to ongoing symptoms.

**Case Example: James's Core Awakening**

James, a 38-year-old construction worker, developed chronic low back pain after a workplace injury. Despite undergoing physical therapy and trying various treatments, his pain persisted. He struggled with unpredictable pain flares that interfered with work and family activities.

His physical therapist recommended Pilates as an adjunct to traditional treatment. James was initially resistant, viewing Pilates as "too gentle" for his condition. However, he agreed to try several sessions to see if it might help.

The Pilates instructor began with basic exercises designed to activate his deep core muscles. James was surprised by how challenging these seemingly simple movements were. He realized that his "core strength" from construction work didn't translate to the stability and control required for proper spinal function.

The program progressed gradually, adding complexity and challenge as James's control improved. He learned to engage his core muscles during everyday activities, reducing stress on his spine. The precise, controlled nature of Pilates movements helped him develop better body awareness and movement quality.

After three months of regular Pilates practice, James experienced significant improvements in pain intensity and functional capacity. He had fewer pain flares and felt more confident in his ability to manage his condition. His case demonstrates how Pilates can complement traditional physical therapy by addressing movement quality and core stability.

**Creating Your Personal Movement Plan**

Developing an effective movement plan requires careful consideration of your specific condition, capabilities, and preferences. The most effective program is one that you'll actually follow consistently, which means it must be realistic, enjoyable, and adaptable to your lifestyle.

## Assessment and Goal Setting

The first step in creating your movement plan involves honest assessment of your current capabilities and limitations. This assessment should include physical factors like strength, flexibility, and endurance, as well as psychological factors like fear-avoidance behaviors and self-efficacy.

Goal setting should follow the SMART criteria: Specific, Measurable, Achievable, Relevant, and Time-bound. Goals should focus on function and quality of life rather than just pain reduction. For example, "I will walk for 20 minutes three times per week" is more effective than "I will reduce my pain."

## Progression Principles

Successful movement programs follow specific progression principles that minimize the risk of symptom flares while promoting steady improvement. The most important principle is gradual progression - increasing intensity, duration, or complexity slowly over time.

The 10% rule provides a useful guideline: increase activity by no more than 10% per week. This approach allows tissues to adapt while minimizing the risk of overuse injuries or pain flares. If symptoms increase, the progression may be too aggressive and should be slowed.

## Integration with Daily Life

The most successful movement programs integrate seamlessly with daily life rather than requiring significant lifestyle changes. This might involve taking stairs instead of elevators, parking farther away, or incorporating movement breaks into the workday.

Activity pacing represents a crucial skill for people with chronic pain. This involves alternating periods of activity with rest, preventing the boom-bust cycle that characterizes many chronic pain conditions.

Pacing allows for consistent activity levels while preventing symptom flares.

## Monitoring and Adjustment

Regular monitoring allows for timely adjustments to your movement plan. This might involve tracking pain levels, activity duration, or functional improvements. The key is identifying patterns that help optimize your program.

Flexibility in your approach is essential. Some days will be better than others, and your program should accommodate these variations. Having both "good day" and "bad day" options ensures that you can maintain some level of activity regardless of how you feel.

## The Path Forward

Movement-based interventions represent the foundation of effective pain management. The evidence consistently demonstrates that appropriate physical activity can reduce pain intensity, improve function, and enhance quality of life across multiple pain conditions. However, success requires more than just knowing what to do - it requires understanding how to implement these strategies safely and effectively.

The key to successful movement therapy lies in finding the right balance between challenge and safety. Too little activity fails to produce beneficial adaptations, while too much activity can worsen symptoms and reinforce fear-avoidance behaviors. This balance is individual and may require professional guidance to achieve.

The next chapter will explore hands-on healing modalities that can complement your movement program. These approaches can help address specific impairments, reduce pain, and improve movement quality, creating a comprehensive approach to pain management.

## Practical Wisdom

Movement is medicine, but like any medicine, it must be prescribed and administered correctly. The most sophisticated exercise program won't help if you can't or won't follow it consistently. Start small, progress gradually, and focus on building habits that can be maintained long-term.

Your body has an remarkable capacity for adaptation and healing. By providing it with appropriate movement challenges, you can stimulate positive changes that reduce pain and improve function. The journey may be gradual, but the destination - a life where pain doesn't control your activities - is worth the effort.

**Essential Principles for Movement Success:**

- Physical therapy provides the foundation for evidence-based movement interventions

- Aerobic exercise offers powerful pain-relieving benefits when properly prescribed and progressed

- Yoga and tai chi combine physical movement with mental training for comprehensive pain management

- Pilates addresses core stability and movement quality, particularly beneficial for spinal conditions

- Personal movement plans must be realistic, enjoyable, and adaptable to individual needs and capabilities

- Gradual progression prevents symptom flares while promoting steady improvement

# Chapter 5: Hands-On Healing Modalities

The human touch has healing power that extends far beyond simple comfort. When applied skillfully by trained practitioners, manual therapies can reduce pain, improve function, and accelerate recovery in ways that complement movement-based interventions. These hands-on approaches work through multiple mechanisms, from direct effects on tissues to complex neurological responses that alter pain processing.

Understanding how these modalities work - and how to choose appropriate practitioners - empowers you to make informed decisions about incorporating them into your pain management plan. The key lies in recognizing that effective manual therapy requires both technical skill and clinical reasoning to address your specific needs and conditions.

## Acupuncture Demystified

Acupuncture has transitioned from alternative medicine to mainstream healthcare based on robust scientific evidence. The American College of Physicians now includes acupuncture in its clinical practice guidelines for chronic low back pain, recognizing its effectiveness for pain management (17). This endorsement reflects decades of research demonstrating acupuncture's benefits for various pain conditions.

The practice involves inserting thin needles into specific points on the body to stimulate healing responses. While the traditional explanations involving energy meridians may seem foreign to Western thinking, modern research has identified clear physiological mechanisms that explain acupuncture's effectiveness.

## How Acupuncture Works

Acupuncture works through multiple mechanisms that affect pain processing at local, spinal, and brain levels. Locally, needle insertion stimulates nerve endings and triggers the release of various chemicals that reduce inflammation and promote healing. At the spinal level, acupuncture activates the gate control mechanism, reducing pain signal transmission to the brain.

Perhaps most importantly, acupuncture stimulates the release of endorphins and other neurotransmitters that provide natural pain relief. Brain imaging studies show that acupuncture treatment activates regions associated with pain regulation while reducing activity in areas that process pain sensations.

The needling technique itself influences treatment outcomes. Skilled practitioners can manipulate needles to produce specific sensations and physiological responses. This technical expertise, combined with proper point selection, determines treatment effectiveness.

**Case Example: Patricia's Migraine Relief**

Patricia, a 42-year-old marketing executive, had suffered from chronic migraines for over a decade. Her headaches occurred 15-20 days per month, significantly impacting her work performance and family life. Traditional treatments provided minimal relief while causing troublesome side effects.

Her neurologist recommended acupuncture as an adjunct to her medical treatment. Patricia was initially skeptical, viewing acupuncture as unscientific. However, the mounting research evidence and her doctor's endorsement convinced her to try.

The acupuncturist began with a comprehensive assessment that included not only her headache patterns but also her sleep, stress levels, and overall health. The treatment plan involved weekly sessions for eight weeks, with specific acupuncture points selected based on her individual presentation.

During the first session, Patricia experienced immediate relaxation and a sense of calm she hadn't felt in years. The needles were barely perceptible, and she found the experience surprisingly pleasant. More importantly, she noticed that her headache intensity decreased following each treatment.

By the fourth week, Patricia's headache frequency had decreased from 15-20 days per month to 8-10 days. The headaches that did occur were less intense and more responsive to her usual medications. After completing the initial treatment series, she continued with monthly maintenance sessions.

Six months later, Patricia's headache frequency had stabilized at 3-5 days per month - a 75% reduction from her baseline. She was able to reduce her preventive medications while maintaining better pain control. Her case demonstrates how acupuncture can provide significant relief for conditions that respond poorly to conventional treatments.

## Research Supporting Acupuncture

Multiple systematic reviews have examined acupuncture's effectiveness for pain management. A comprehensive analysis published in the Archives of Internal Medicine found that acupuncture was superior to both sham acupuncture and usual care for chronic pain conditions (18). The effects were clinically meaningful and persisted for months after treatment completion.

The evidence is particularly strong for certain conditions. Acupuncture shows consistent benefits for chronic low back pain, neck pain, osteoarthritis, and headaches. The American College of Physicians specifically recommends acupuncture for chronic low back pain based on this evidence (19).

Quality matters significantly in acupuncture research. Studies using proper controls and adequate treatment doses show larger effect sizes than those with weaker methodologies. This pattern suggests that acupuncture's benefits are real and can be optimized through skilled practice.

## Massage Therapy Techniques

Massage therapy encompasses a wide range of techniques designed to manipulate soft tissues for therapeutic benefit. Far from being a luxury spa treatment, therapeutic massage is a legitimate medical intervention with documented benefits for pain management and functional improvement.

The American College of Physicians includes massage therapy in its recommendations for chronic low back pain treatment (20). This endorsement reflects growing recognition of massage therapy's role in evidence-based pain management.

**Types of Therapeutic Massage**

Different massage techniques serve different purposes and are appropriate for different conditions. Swedish massage uses long, flowing strokes to promote relaxation and improve circulation. Deep tissue massage targets deeper muscle layers to address chronic tension and adhesions. Trigger point therapy focuses on specific areas of muscle hyperactivity that refer pain to other locations.

The choice of technique should be based on your specific condition and treatment goals. A skilled massage therapist will assess your needs and select appropriate techniques, often combining multiple approaches within a single session.

**Case Example: Michael's Recovery Journey**

Michael, a 55-year-old software engineer, developed chronic neck and shoulder pain after years of computer work. His pain was constant and interfered with both work and sleep. Physical therapy had provided some benefit, but significant muscle tension remained.

His physical therapist recommended massage therapy to address persistent muscle tension that was limiting his progress. Michael was initially hesitant, viewing massage as something for relaxation rather than medical treatment. However, he agreed to try therapeutic massage as part of his treatment plan.

The massage therapist began with a comprehensive assessment that identified specific areas of muscle tension and trigger points. The treatment plan involved weekly sessions focusing on the neck, shoulders, and upper back. The therapist used a combination of

Swedish massage for relaxation and trigger point therapy for specific problem areas.

During the first session, Michael experienced immediate relief from muscle tension. The massage therapist identified several trigger points that were contributing to his pain pattern. Treatment of these points provided relief that extended beyond the massage session.

Over six weeks of treatment, Michael noticed progressive improvement in his pain levels and range of motion. The massage therapy helped maintain the gains he made during physical therapy while addressing residual muscle tension. His sleep improved, and he was able to work more comfortably.

Michael's case illustrates how massage therapy can complement other treatments by addressing specific impairments. The combination of massage therapy and physical therapy provided better outcomes than either treatment alone.

**Mechanisms of Massage Therapy**

Massage therapy works through multiple mechanisms that affect both local tissues and systemic responses. Locally, massage improves blood flow, reduces muscle tension, and promotes tissue flexibility. These effects can directly reduce pain and improve function.

Systemically, massage activates the parasympathetic nervous system, promoting relaxation and reducing stress hormones. This response can break the cycle of pain and muscle tension that characterizes many chronic conditions. Massage also stimulates the release of endorphins, providing natural pain relief.

The pressure and movement used in massage can activate the gate control mechanism, reducing pain signal transmission to the brain. This effect explains why massage often provides immediate pain relief that can last for hours or days after treatment.

**Chiropractic and Osteopathy**

Chiropractic and osteopathic manipulative treatment focus on the relationship between spinal alignment and overall health. These approaches use manual techniques to address joint dysfunction and improve movement patterns. While controversial in some circles, research supports their effectiveness for certain pain conditions.

The key to understanding these treatments lies in recognizing that they address mechanical dysfunction rather than attempting to cure diseases through spinal adjustment. Modern evidence-based practitioners focus on improving joint mobility and reducing pain rather than making broad health claims.

## Chiropractic Care for Pain Management

Chiropractic treatment involves manual manipulation of spinal joints to improve mobility and reduce pain. The approach is based on the principle that joint dysfunction can contribute to pain and that restoring normal joint function can provide relief.

Research supports chiropractic care for certain conditions, particularly acute and chronic low back pain. A systematic review found that spinal manipulation provides short-term relief for low back pain and may be as effective as other common treatments (21).

The effectiveness of chiropractic care depends largely on proper patient selection and skilled application. Conditions involving joint dysfunction and mechanical pain are most likely to respond to manipulative treatment. Inflammatory conditions or those involving nerve compression may require different approaches.

## Case Example: David's Back Pain Success

David, a 35-year-old warehouse worker, developed acute low back pain after lifting a heavy box. The pain was severe and localized to one side of his lower back. Movement was limited, and he had difficulty performing basic activities.

His primary care physician referred him to a chiropractor for evaluation and treatment. The chiropractor's assessment revealed restricted movement in several lumbar joints along with muscle spasm. The treatment plan included spinal manipulation, soft tissue techniques, and home exercises.

The first treatment provided immediate relief from David's acute pain. The manipulation restored normal joint movement while soft tissue techniques addressed muscle spasm. David was able to move more freely and experienced significant pain reduction.

Treatment continued twice weekly for two weeks, then weekly for another month. Each session included manipulation, soft tissue work, and progression of exercises. David gradually returned to full activity while maintaining his improvement.

David's case demonstrates how chiropractic care can be effective for acute mechanical back pain. The combination of manipulation and exercise provided rapid relief while preventing chronicity. His success illustrates the importance of proper patient selection and skilled treatment.

## Osteopathic Manipulative Treatment

Osteopathic manipulative treatment (OMT) uses manual techniques to address dysfunction in the musculoskeletal system. Osteopathic physicians receive specialized training in these techniques, which they integrate with conventional medical practice.

OMT encompasses a wide range of techniques, from gentle mobilization to high-velocity manipulation. The approach is individualized based on the patient's condition and the physician's assessment findings. Treatment goals focus on improving function and reducing pain rather than correcting supposed "subluxations."

Research supports OMT for certain conditions, particularly low back pain and neck pain. The evidence suggests that OMT can provide pain relief and functional improvement comparable to other manual therapy approaches.

## Myofascial Release

Myofascial release targets the fascial system - the connective tissue network that surrounds and connects muscles throughout the body. This approach recognizes that restrictions in fascial tissue can contribute to pain and dysfunction, requiring specialized techniques for effective treatment.

The fascial system plays a crucial role in movement and posture. Restrictions in this system can create patterns of dysfunction that affect multiple body regions. Myofascial release techniques aim to restore normal fascial mobility and reduce pain.


**Understanding Fascial Dysfunction**

Fascial restrictions can develop following injury, surgery, or repetitive stress. These restrictions can create tension patterns that affect movement and contribute to pain. The interconnected nature of the fascial system means that restrictions in one area can affect distant regions.

Myofascial release techniques use sustained pressure and stretching to address these restrictions. The approach requires skilled assessment to identify restriction patterns and appropriate treatment techniques. Treatment is typically slower and more sustained than traditional massage techniques.

**Case Example: Jennifer's Fascial Recovery**

Jennifer, a 29-year-old dancer, developed chronic hip and leg pain following a fall. Despite extensive medical evaluation, no specific injury was identified. Traditional treatments provided minimal relief, and she was unable to return to dancing.

A physical therapist specialized in myofascial release evaluated Jennifer and identified extensive fascial restrictions throughout her hip and leg. These restrictions were creating movement dysfunction and pain that hadn't responded to conventional treatment.

Treatment involved sustained pressure applied to specific fascial restrictions. The techniques were gentle but required prolonged application to achieve fascial release. Jennifer initially found the treatment uncomfortable but noticed immediate improvement in her movement.

Over several months of treatment, Jennifer experienced progressive improvement in her pain and movement quality. The myofascial release addressed restrictions that hadn't been identified through conventional assessment. She was eventually able to return to dancing at her previous level.

Jennifer's case demonstrates how myofascial release can address problems that don't respond to conventional treatment. The specialized assessment and treatment techniques provided relief when other approaches had failed.

## Choosing the Right Practitioner

The effectiveness of manual therapy depends heavily on practitioner skill and experience. Choosing the right practitioner requires understanding their training, expertise, and approach to treatment. This decision can significantly impact your treatment outcomes and overall experience.

## Credentials and Training

Different manual therapy practitioners have varying levels of training and scope of practice. Physical therapists receive comprehensive training in musculoskeletal disorders and movement dysfunction. Massage therapists complete specialized training in soft tissue techniques. Chiropractors focus on spinal manipulation and joint dysfunction.

Licensing requirements vary by state and profession. All legitimate practitioners should be licensed in their respective fields and able to provide evidence of their credentials. Additional certifications in specialized techniques may indicate advanced training and expertise.

## Treatment Philosophy and Approach

Different practitioners may have varying philosophies about pain and treatment. Evidence-based practitioners focus on techniques supported by research and integrate their treatments with conventional medical care. Others may emphasize alternative theories or make claims not supported by scientific evidence.

The best practitioners combine technical skill with clinical reasoning. They should be able to explain their assessment findings, treatment rationale, and expected outcomes. They should also be willing to communicate with your other healthcare providers and modify their approach based on your response.

**Questions to Ask Potential Practitioners**

Before beginning treatment, ask about the practitioner's experience with your specific condition. How many patients with similar problems have they treated? What outcomes do they typically achieve? How do they determine if treatment is working?

Ask about their treatment approach and what to expect during sessions. How many treatments are typically needed? What will you do during treatment? What should you expect to feel during and after treatment?

Communication style is important for successful treatment. The practitioner should listen to your concerns, explain procedures clearly, and involve you in treatment decisions. They should also be willing to answer questions and adjust their approach based on your feedback.

**Integration with Other Treatments**

Manual therapy works best when integrated with other evidence-based treatments. These approaches can complement exercise programs, address specific impairments, and accelerate recovery. The key is coordinating care to ensure treatments work together rather than at cross-purposes.

Communication between practitioners is essential for optimal outcomes. Your physical therapist, massage therapist, and chiropractor should understand each other's treatment goals and approaches. This coordination prevents conflicting advice and ensures treatments complement each other.

The timing of different treatments can affect outcomes. Some manual therapies may be more effective when performed before exercise, while others may be better afterward. Your practitioners should coordinate timing to optimize treatment effects.

**Clinical Perspectives**

Manual therapy represents a valuable component of comprehensive pain management. These approaches can address specific impairments, reduce pain, and improve function when applied skillfully by qualified practitioners. The key is understanding what each approach can and cannot do, and how they fit into your overall treatment plan.

The evidence supporting manual therapy continues to grow, with research identifying specific conditions and patient populations that benefit most from these approaches. This evidence-based approach helps ensure that manual therapy is used appropriately and effectively.

The next chapter will explore technology-enhanced approaches to pain relief. These innovative treatments offer new possibilities for pain management while complementing traditional manual therapy approaches.

**Key Insights for Manual Therapy Success:**

- Acupuncture provides scientifically validated pain relief through multiple neurological mechanisms

- Massage therapy addresses soft tissue dysfunction and promotes relaxation responses that reduce pain

- Chiropractic and osteopathic treatments can effectively address mechanical joint dysfunction

- Myofascial release targets the fascial system to address movement restrictions and pain patterns

- Practitioner selection significantly impacts treatment outcomes and requires careful consideration

- Integration with other treatments optimizes manual therapy benefits and improves overall outcomes

# Chapter 6: Technology-Enhanced Pain Relief

The intersection of technology and pain management has produced remarkable innovations that extend far beyond traditional treatments. These technological advances offer new possibilities for pain relief while making existing treatments more accessible and effective. From electrical stimulation devices you can use at home to virtual reality systems that transport you away from pain, technology is revolutionizing how we approach pain management.

Understanding these technological options empowers you to make informed decisions about incorporating them into your pain management plan. The key lies in recognizing that technology should complement, not replace, fundamental approaches like movement and manual therapy.

## TENS Units and Electrical Stimulation

Transcutaneous electrical nerve stimulation (TENS) represents one of the most accessible and well-researched technological approaches to pain management. These devices deliver controlled electrical impulses through electrodes placed on the skin, activating pain-relieving mechanisms in the nervous system.

The CDC includes TENS therapy in its recommendations for non-opioid pain management approaches (22). This endorsement reflects decades of research demonstrating TENS effectiveness for various pain conditions. The treatment is particularly appealing because it's non-invasive, has minimal side effects, and can be used at home.

## How TENS Works

TENS devices work primarily through the gate control mechanism described in earlier chapters. The electrical stimulation activates large-diameter nerve fibers that can "close the gate" on pain signals traveling to the brain. This mechanism explains why TENS often provides immediate pain relief during and shortly after treatment.

The electrical stimulation also triggers the release of endorphins, the body's natural pain-relieving chemicals. This effect can provide longer-lasting pain relief that extends beyond the stimulation period. The combination of gate control and endorphin release makes TENS effective for both acute and chronic pain conditions.

Different stimulation parameters produce different effects. High-frequency stimulation (above 80 Hz) primarily activates the gate control mechanism, providing immediate but short-lasting relief. Low-frequency stimulation (below 10 Hz) triggers endorphin release, producing longer-lasting but delayed pain relief.

**Case Example: Carol's Arthritis Management**

Carol, a 68-year-old retired teacher, developed severe osteoarthritis in her knees that significantly limited her mobility. Walking became painful, and she found herself becoming increasingly sedentary. Traditional pain medications provided some relief but caused stomach upset and made her feel drowsy.

Her physical therapist recommended a TENS unit as an adjunct to her treatment program. Carol was initially skeptical about the small, battery-powered device, questioning how such a simple-looking apparatus could provide meaningful pain relief.

The physical therapist taught Carol how to position the electrodes around her knee joints and adjust the stimulation settings. During the first session, Carol experienced immediate reduction in her knee pain. The electrical sensation was mildly tingling but not uncomfortable, and she could clearly feel the difference in her pain levels.

Carol began using the TENS unit for 30 minutes twice daily, typically during her morning routine and while watching television in the evening. The device provided consistent pain relief that allowed her to be more active throughout the day. She was able to reduce her pain medication use while maintaining better function.

After three months of regular TENS use, Carol reported a 50% reduction in average pain intensity. More importantly, she was able to resume walking for exercise and participate in activities she had previously avoided. Her case demonstrates how TENS can provide meaningful pain relief while supporting increased activity levels.

## Optimizing TENS Treatment

Successful TENS treatment requires proper electrode placement, appropriate stimulation parameters, and consistent use. Electrode placement should target the area of pain or the nerve pathways that supply the painful region. The stimulation intensity should be strong enough to produce a comfortable tingling sensation without causing muscle contractions.

Treatment duration and frequency can be adjusted based on individual response and needs. Some people benefit from brief, frequent sessions, while others prefer longer, less frequent treatments. The device can be used as needed for pain control or on a regular schedule for more consistent relief.

## Other Forms of Electrical Stimulation

Beyond TENS, several other forms of electrical stimulation offer pain relief benefits. Interferential current therapy uses medium-frequency electrical stimulation to penetrate deeper tissues. This approach can be effective for deeper pain conditions that don't respond well to TENS.

Electrical muscle stimulation (EMS) targets muscle tissue directly, causing muscle contractions that can improve circulation and reduce pain. This approach is particularly useful for conditions involving muscle weakness or disuse atrophy.

Percutaneous electrical nerve stimulation (PENS) combines principles of TENS and acupuncture by delivering electrical stimulation through acupuncture needles. This approach may be more effective than surface electrode stimulation for certain conditions.

## Virtual Reality for Pain Management

Virtual reality (VR) technology has emerged as a powerful tool for pain management, working through distraction and immersion to reduce pain perception. Research published in BMC Medicine and PubMed Central has documented significant pain reduction benefits across various conditions and treatment settings (23, 24).

VR pain management works by engaging multiple sensory systems simultaneously, creating an immersive experience that redirects attention away from pain. This distraction effect can be so powerful that it allows medical procedures to be performed with reduced need for pain medication.

### The Science of VR Pain Relief

VR affects pain perception through several mechanisms. The primary effect is attentional distraction - the brain has limited capacity to process information, and engaging visual, auditory, and sometimes tactile senses through VR leaves less capacity for processing pain signals.

Brain imaging studies show that VR treatment reduces activity in pain-processing regions while increasing activity in areas associated with attention and sensory processing. These changes correspond to reported reductions in pain intensity and unpleasantness.

The immersive nature of VR creates a sense of presence that can be more effective than traditional distraction techniques. Users report feeling transported to the virtual environment, creating psychological distance from their pain experience.

### Case Example: Mark's Burn Recovery

Mark, a 34-year-old construction worker, suffered severe burns on his hands and arms in a workplace accident. The daily wound care procedures were extremely painful, requiring high doses of pain medication that left him drowsy and nauseous. The medical team sought alternatives to reduce his suffering during treatment.

The burn center introduced VR therapy during wound care procedures. Mark wore a VR headset that transported him to a snowy mountain environment where he could throw snowballs at virtual targets. The cold, peaceful environment provided psychological contrast to the painful medical procedures.

During his first VR session, Mark reported significant reduction in pain intensity during wound care. The immersive environment captured his attention so completely that he was surprised when the procedure ended. He requested VR for all subsequent treatments.

Over two weeks of daily wound care with VR, Mark's pain medication requirements decreased by 60%. He experienced less anxiety about treatments and reported better sleep quality. The VR system allowed him to participate actively in his pain management while reducing his dependence on medications.

Mark's case demonstrates how VR can provide meaningful pain relief during medical procedures. The technology offered benefits that extended beyond the treatment sessions, improving his overall experience and recovery.

### VR Applications for Chronic Pain

Virtual reality shows promise for chronic pain management beyond acute medical procedures. VR programs designed for chronic pain typically combine distraction with relaxation training, mindfulness exercises, and education about pain management.

Some VR programs use biofeedback to create interactive experiences that respond to the user's physiological state. These systems can teach relaxation techniques while providing immediate feedback about stress levels and pain responses.

The accessibility of VR technology continues to improve, with smartphone-based systems making VR pain management more affordable and convenient. These developments may make VR pain management accessible to broader populations of people with chronic pain.

## Neuromodulation Devices

Neuromodulation represents the most advanced technological approach to pain management, using electrical or magnetic stimulation to modify nervous system activity. These devices can provide significant pain relief for conditions that don't respond to conventional treatments.

Research published in PubMed Central has documented the effectiveness of various neuromodulation approaches for chronic pain conditions (25, 26, 27, 28). These treatments offer hope for people with severe, treatment-resistant pain conditions.

## Spinal Cord Stimulation

Spinal cord stimulation (SCS) involves implanting electrodes near the spinal cord to deliver electrical stimulation that modifies pain signals. This approach can provide significant pain relief for certain types of chronic pain, particularly neuropathic pain conditions.

The procedure involves two stages: a trial period with temporary electrodes to assess effectiveness, followed by permanent implantation if the trial is successful. The stimulation parameters can be adjusted to optimize pain relief while minimizing side effects.

Modern SCS systems offer sophisticated programming options that can target specific pain patterns. Some systems use closed-loop technology that adjusts stimulation based on the patient's activity level and pain patterns.

## Case Example: Susan's Neuropathic Pain Relief

Susan, a 51-year-old nurse, developed complex regional pain syndrome (CRPS) following a minor ankle injury. Her pain was severe, burning, and constant, affecting her entire lower leg. Traditional treatments including medications, physical therapy, and nerve blocks provided minimal relief.

After two years of unsuccessful treatments, Susan's pain specialist recommended spinal cord stimulation. The procedure involved placing electrodes in the epidural space near her spinal cord. During the trial period, Susan experienced 70% reduction in pain intensity.

The permanent implantation was performed as an outpatient procedure. The device was programmed to deliver stimulation that produced a comfortable tingling sensation over her painful area. Susan could adjust the stimulation using a handheld controller.

With the spinal cord stimulator, Susan was able to reduce her pain medication use by 80% while maintaining better pain control. She returned to work part-time and resumed many activities she had abandoned due to pain. Her case demonstrates how neuromodulation can provide relief for severe, treatment-resistant pain conditions.

**Peripheral Nerve Stimulation**

Peripheral nerve stimulation (PNS) targets specific peripheral nerves rather than the spinal cord. This approach can be effective for localized pain conditions and may be less invasive than spinal cord stimulation.

PNS devices can be implanted surgically or placed temporarily for specific conditions. The stimulation parameters are adjusted to provide optimal pain relief while minimizing side effects. Some newer systems use wireless technology to reduce complications associated with implanted leads.

**Transcranial Magnetic Stimulation**

Transcranial magnetic stimulation (TMS) uses magnetic fields to stimulate specific brain regions involved in pain processing. This non-invasive approach can be effective for certain types of chronic pain, particularly when psychological factors play a significant role.

TMS treatment typically involves multiple sessions over several weeks. The magnetic stimulation is delivered through a coil placed on the scalp, targeting specific brain regions associated with pain processing and mood regulation.

## Heat and Cold Therapy

Heat and cold therapy represent simple but effective technological approaches to pain management. These treatments work through different mechanisms and are appropriate for different types of pain conditions.

The American College of Physicians includes heat and cold therapy in its recommendations for acute and chronic pain management (29, 30). These treatments are particularly appealing because they're safe, accessible, and can be used at home.

### Heat Therapy Mechanisms

Heat therapy works through several mechanisms that can provide pain relief. Heat increases blood flow to treated areas, promoting healing and reducing muscle tension. The thermal stimulation can also activate the gate control mechanism, reducing pain signal transmission.

Heat therapy is particularly effective for chronic pain conditions involving muscle tension and stiffness. The increased blood flow can help deliver nutrients and remove metabolic waste products that contribute to pain and dysfunction.

### Case Example: Robert's Muscle Spasm Relief

Robert, a 47-year-old truck driver, developed chronic muscle spasms in his neck and shoulders due to prolonged driving and poor posture. The spasms were painful and limited his range of motion, affecting both his work performance and sleep quality.

His physical therapist recommended heat therapy as part of his treatment program. Robert began using a heating pad for 20 minutes before his exercise sessions and again in the evening before bed. The heat provided immediate relief from muscle tension and made his exercises more comfortable.

Robert also used heat therapy during long driving shifts, using a portable heating pad designed for vehicle use. The heat helped prevent muscle tension from building up during extended periods of driving.

After several weeks of regular heat therapy, Robert reported significant improvement in his muscle tension and pain levels. He was able to sleep better and felt more comfortable during long drives. The heat therapy complemented his exercise program and helped maintain his improvements.

**Cold Therapy Applications**

Cold therapy works through different mechanisms than heat and is appropriate for different conditions. Cold reduces inflammation, numbs pain, and can help control swelling. It's particularly effective for acute injuries and inflammatory conditions.

Cold therapy can be delivered through various methods, from simple ice packs to sophisticated cooling systems. The key is controlling the temperature and duration of treatment to maximize benefits while preventing tissue damage.

Contrast therapy, alternating between heat and cold, can be effective for certain conditions. This approach can improve circulation while providing pain relief through multiple mechanisms.

**Emerging Technologies**

The field of pain management technology continues to evolve rapidly, with new innovations constantly emerging. These developments offer hope for more effective, accessible, and personalized pain management approaches.

Wearable devices are becoming increasingly sophisticated, offering continuous monitoring of pain-related parameters and delivering treatments as needed. These devices can provide real-time feedback about activity levels, stress, and pain patterns.

Artificial intelligence is being integrated into pain management devices to provide personalized treatment recommendations. These systems can analyze individual response patterns and adjust treatments automatically for optimal outcomes.

Smartphone applications are expanding access to pain management tools, providing everything from guided meditation to exercise programs. These apps can make evidence-based pain management techniques more accessible and convenient.

## The Future of Pain Technology

Technology will continue to play an increasingly important role in pain management, offering new possibilities for relief and recovery. The key is using these tools appropriately as part of a comprehensive pain management plan that includes movement, manual therapy, and lifestyle modifications.

The most promising developments combine technological innovation with evidence-based practice, creating tools that are both effective and accessible. As these technologies continue to evolve, they will provide new options for people seeking relief from chronic pain.

The next chapter will explore mind-body approaches to pain management, examining how psychological and cognitive techniques can complement the technological and physical approaches we've discussed.

## Technology Integration Strategies

Technology-enhanced pain relief offers powerful tools for managing chronic pain when used appropriately. These approaches work best when integrated with traditional treatments and lifestyle modifications. The key is understanding how different technologies can address specific aspects of your pain experience while supporting your overall management plan.

Success with technological approaches requires realistic expectations and consistent use. Like any treatment, these tools work best when used as part of a comprehensive approach that addresses multiple aspects of chronic pain. The combination of technology with movement, manual therapy, and lifestyle changes can provide synergistic benefits that exceed what any single approach can achieve.

**Essential Technology Applications:**

- TENS units provide accessible, home-based pain relief through electrical stimulation

- Virtual reality offers powerful distraction-based pain management during procedures and daily activities

- Neuromodulation devices can provide significant relief for severe, treatment-resistant pain conditions

- Heat and cold therapy remain simple but effective tools for managing various pain conditions

- Emerging technologies continue to expand options for personalized, accessible pain management

- Integration with traditional treatments optimizes technological approaches for comprehensive pain management

# Chapter 7: Harnessing Your Mind's Pain-Fighting Power

The brain you carry in your skull is the most sophisticated pain management system ever created. This three-pound organ processes every pain signal you experience, determines its meaning, and decides how intensely you'll feel it. More remarkably, your brain can learn to reduce pain through specific mental training techniques that are as measurable and reproducible as any medication.

The misconception that psychological pain treatments address "imaginary" pain has hindered many people from accessing these powerful tools. The reality is that mind-body approaches work by changing actual brain chemistry and neural pathways. Brain scans show that psychological interventions produce real, measurable changes in pain-processing regions - changes that correspond directly to reported improvements in pain intensity and quality of life.

## Cognitive Behavioral Therapy for Pain

Cognitive Behavioral Therapy for Pain (CBT-P) represents the most researched and effective psychological approach to pain management. This structured treatment focuses on identifying and changing thoughts, feelings, and behaviors that contribute to pain and suffering. The Cleveland Clinic Journal of Medicine has published extensive research documenting CBT-P's effectiveness across numerous pain conditions (31).

CBT-P works on a simple but powerful principle: your thoughts about pain directly influence how much pain you experience. This doesn't mean pain is "all in your head" - it means your brain's interpretation of pain signals can be modified through systematic training.

The approach differs significantly from traditional talk therapy. CBT-P is structured, goal-oriented, and skills-based. Sessions focus on learning specific techniques rather than exploring past experiences. The treatment typically involves 8-16 sessions over several months, with homework assignments to practice new skills.

## How CBT-P Changes Pain Processing

CBT-P works through several mechanisms that directly affect pain perception. The treatment helps identify catastrophic thinking patterns - thoughts like "this pain will never end" or "I can't handle this" - that amplify pain signals. By replacing these thoughts with more realistic, balanced perspectives, people can reduce their pain intensity.

The therapy also addresses fear-avoidance behaviors that often develop with chronic pain. Many people begin avoiding activities they associate with pain, leading to physical deconditioning and increased pain sensitivity. CBT-P helps people gradually return to meaningful activities while managing their anxiety about pain.

Stress and anxiety directly increase pain sensitivity through measurable changes in brain chemistry. CBT-P teaches relaxation techniques and stress management skills that can reduce these physiological responses, creating a calmer internal environment that processes pain less intensely.

## Case Example: Sarah's Transformation

Sarah, a 44-year-old marketing manager, developed chronic back pain after a workplace injury. Despite surgery and extensive physical therapy, her pain persisted and gradually worsened. She found herself thinking constantly about her pain, worrying about her future, and avoiding activities she once enjoyed.

Her pain psychologist began CBT-P by helping Sarah identify her thought patterns. She discovered that she consistently catastrophized about her pain, imagining worst-case scenarios and interpreting normal fluctuations as signs of permanent damage. These thoughts created anxiety that made her pain feel more intense.

The therapy focused on teaching Sarah to recognize these unhelpful thoughts and replace them with more balanced perspectives. Instead of thinking "this pain means I'm getting worse," she learned to think "pain fluctuates naturally, and this doesn't mean permanent damage."

Sarah also learned relaxation techniques including progressive muscle relaxation and guided imagery. These skills helped her manage stress and anxiety, which had been amplifying her pain. She practiced these techniques daily, gradually building her confidence in her ability to influence her pain experience.

The behavioral component involved gradually returning to activities she had abandoned due to fear of pain. Sarah started with brief walks and slowly increased her activity level. Each successful experience built her confidence and reduced her fear-avoidance behaviors.

After 12 weeks of CBT-P, Sarah reported a 60% reduction in pain intensity and had returned to most of her previous activities. More importantly, she felt in control of her pain rather than controlled by it. Her case demonstrates how CBT-P can transform the pain experience by addressing the psychological factors that amplify suffering.

**Core CBT-P Techniques**

CBT-P encompasses several specific techniques that can be learned and practiced independently. Thought challenging involves identifying negative thought patterns and examining evidence for and against these thoughts. This process helps develop more balanced, realistic perspectives on pain.

Activity pacing teaches people to balance activity with rest to prevent pain flares while maintaining function. This technique involves breaking large tasks into smaller components and alternating periods of activity with brief rest breaks.

Relaxation training includes various techniques like deep breathing, progressive muscle relaxation, and guided imagery. These skills help activate the body's relaxation response, reducing stress hormones that can amplify pain.

Problem-solving skills help people address practical challenges that chronic pain creates. This might involve workplace accommodations, relationship adjustments, or lifestyle modifications that support pain management.

**Case Example: Michael's Return to Work**

Michael, a 39-year-old teacher, developed chronic neck pain that interfered with his ability to work. He found himself calling in sick frequently and worrying constantly about his job security. His pain seemed to worsen during stressful periods, creating a cycle of pain and anxiety.

CBT-P helped Michael identify the connection between his stress levels and pain intensity. He learned that his worry about work performance was actually making his pain worse, creating a vicious cycle. The therapy taught him stress management techniques and helped him develop more realistic thoughts about his situation.

Michael worked with his therapist to develop a graded return-to-work plan. He started with shorter days and gradually increased his hours as his confidence grew. The therapy also addressed his catastrophic thoughts about job loss, helping him develop more balanced perspectives.

The treatment included communication skills training to help Michael discuss his condition with his supervisor and colleagues. He learned to request appropriate accommodations while maintaining his professional relationships.

After completing CBT-P, Michael was able to return to full-time work with appropriate accommodations. His pain levels had decreased significantly, and he felt confident in his ability to manage flares when they occurred. His case illustrates how CBT-P can address the broader life impacts of chronic pain.

**Mindfulness-Based Stress Reduction**

Mindfulness-Based Stress Reduction (MBSR) offers a structured approach to pain management through meditation and mindfulness practices. Developed by Jon Kabat-Zinn, this eight-week program has been extensively researched and shown to provide significant benefits for chronic pain conditions (32, 33, 34, 35).

MBSR teaches people to observe their pain experience without becoming overwhelmed by it. This approach doesn't aim to eliminate pain but rather to change your relationship with pain. Participants learn to notice pain sensations without automatically reacting with fear, anxiety, or resistance.

The program combines several meditation practices including body scan meditation, sitting meditation, and mindful movement. These practices help develop present-moment awareness and reduce the tendency to ruminate about pain or worry about the future.

**The Eight-Week MBSR Protocol**

The MBSR program follows a structured format that builds skills progressively over eight weeks. Each week introduces new practices while reinforcing previous learning. The program typically involves weekly group sessions lasting 2.5 hours, daily home practice, and one full-day retreat.

Week one introduces the concept of mindfulness and begins with body scan meditation. This practice involves systematically focusing attention on different parts of the body, developing awareness of physical sensations including pain. Participants learn to observe these sensations without judgment or attempts to change them.

Weeks two and three introduce sitting meditation, focusing on breath awareness and expanding attention to include thoughts and emotions. Participants learn to notice when their minds wander to pain-related worries and gently return attention to the present moment.

The middle weeks incorporate mindful movement, including gentle yoga and walking meditation. These practices help people develop a different relationship with their bodies and learn to move mindfully despite pain.

Later weeks focus on integrating mindfulness into daily life, dealing with difficult emotions, and maintaining practice after the program ends. The final sessions emphasize developing a personal practice that can be sustained long-term.

**Case Example: Robert's Mindfulness Journey**

Robert, a 52-year-old accountant, developed chronic fibromyalgia that left him feeling exhausted and in constant pain. He struggled with sleep problems and found himself becoming increasingly irritable with his family. Traditional treatments had provided minimal relief, and he felt desperate for alternatives.

Robert enrolled in an MBSR program with skepticism about meditation. He worried that he wouldn't be able to "quiet his mind" or that the practice would be too difficult given his pain levels. The instructor assured him that mindfulness isn't about stopping thoughts but about changing his relationship with them.

The body scan meditation initially challenged Robert because focusing on his body seemed to intensify his pain awareness. However, the instructor explained that this was normal and that the practice would gradually help him develop a different relationship with pain sensations.

Over several weeks, Robert began to notice subtle changes in his pain experience. He found that when he observed his pain mindfully rather than fighting it, the emotional distress decreased even when the physical sensations remained. This discovery was transformative - he realized that much of his suffering came from his resistance to pain rather than the pain itself.

Robert also learned to use mindfulness during pain flares. Instead of panicking when pain increased, he would use breathing techniques and body awareness to stay grounded in the present moment. This approach helped him manage flares more effectively and reduced his anxiety about pain.

After completing the eight-week program, Robert reported significant improvements in sleep quality, mood, and overall quality of life.

While his pain levels hadn't changed dramatically, his relationship with pain had transformed completely. He continued daily mindfulness practice and felt equipped to handle future challenges.

## Clinical Hypnotherapy

Clinical hypnotherapy for pain management has moved far beyond stage show stereotypes to become a legitimate medical treatment supported by extensive research. Studies published in leading medical journals have documented hypnosis's effectiveness for various pain conditions, with benefits that can equal or exceed those of traditional pain medications (36, 37, 38, 39, 40, 41, 42, 43, 44, 45).

Hypnosis works by accessing altered states of consciousness that allow for direct communication with unconscious processes that influence pain perception. During hypnotic states, people can learn to modify their pain experience through suggestion and imagery.

The process involves inducing a relaxed, focused state of attention that makes people more responsive to therapeutic suggestions. Contrary to popular misconceptions, people remain in control during hypnosis and cannot be forced to do anything against their will.

## Understanding Hypnotic States

Hypnosis represents a naturally occurring altered state of consciousness that people experience regularly. The focused attention while reading a good book, the absorption during a movie, or the automatic driving during a familiar commute all involve hypnotic-like states.

Clinical hypnosis uses these natural capacities therapeutically. The hypnotic state allows for increased suggestibility, making it easier to accept new ideas about pain and healing. It also provides access to unconscious resources that can influence pain perception.

Brain imaging studies show that hypnosis produces measurable changes in pain-processing regions. These changes correspond to reported reductions in pain intensity and unpleasantness. The alterations appear to affect how pain signals are interpreted rather than blocking them entirely.

## Case Example: Linda's Migraine Management

Linda, a 36-year-old nurse, suffered from severe migraines that occurred several times weekly. The headaches were debilitating, forcing her to miss work and avoid social activities. Medications provided some relief but caused side effects that affected her quality of life.

Her pain specialist referred her to a clinical hypnotherapist who specialized in headache treatment. Linda was initially skeptical, associating hypnosis with entertainment rather than medical treatment. The therapist explained the scientific basis for hypnotic pain relief and addressed her concerns about losing control.

The first session involved teaching Linda to enter a hypnotic state through progressive relaxation and focused attention. She was surprised by how pleasant and natural the experience felt. The therapist then used suggestions to help her brain process pain signals differently.

Linda learned self-hypnosis techniques that she could use when she felt a migraine beginning. The approach involved entering a relaxed state and using specific imagery to reduce pain intensity. She practiced these techniques daily, gradually building her skill and confidence.

The hypnotherapy also addressed triggers that seemed to precipitate her migraines. Through hypnotic suggestions, Linda learned to respond differently to stress and to maintain better sleep patterns. These changes helped reduce the frequency of her headaches.

After eight weeks of hypnotherapy, Linda's migraine frequency had decreased by 70%. The headaches that did occur were less intense and more responsive to her self-hypnosis techniques. She was able to reduce her medication use while maintaining better pain control.

**Hypnotic Techniques for Pain**

Several specific hypnotic techniques have proven effective for pain management. Direct suggestion involves telling the unconscious mind to reduce pain intensity or eliminate pain from specific body regions. This straightforward approach can be surprisingly effective for responsive individuals.

Imagery techniques use visualization to modify pain perception. People might imagine pain as a color that gradually fades, or visualize healing energy flowing to painful areas. These images can produce measurable changes in pain intensity and brain activity.

Dissociation techniques help people mentally separate from their pain experience. This might involve imagining themselves outside their body or focusing attention away from painful sensations. These approaches can provide significant relief during acute pain episodes.

Time distortion involves altering the perception of time during painful experiences. People can learn to make brief pain episodes feel longer or make extended painful procedures feel shorter. This technique is particularly useful during medical procedures.

**Biofeedback Training**

Biofeedback training teaches people to control physiological processes that influence pain perception. By providing real-time information about normally unconscious body functions, biofeedback helps people learn to modify muscle tension, heart rate, and other factors that affect pain intensity.

The Cleveland Clinic describes biofeedback as a technique that uses electronic monitoring to convey information about physiological processes (46, 47). This information allows people to learn conscious control over typically automatic functions.

The approach works by making unconscious processes visible through electronic monitoring. People can see their muscle tension levels, heart rate variability, or brain wave patterns on a computer screen. This feedback allows them to experiment with different mental and physical techniques to achieve desired changes.

## Types of Biofeedback for Pain

Electromyographic (EMG) biofeedback monitors muscle tension and is particularly useful for pain conditions involving muscle spasm or tension. People can learn to recognize and reduce muscle tension that contributes to their pain.

Heart rate variability biofeedback teaches people to control their autonomic nervous system responses. This training can help reduce stress and anxiety that amplify pain while promoting relaxation responses that reduce pain intensity.

Neurofeedback monitors brain wave activity and can help people learn to produce brain states associated with relaxation and pain relief. This approach may be particularly beneficial for people whose pain is influenced by stress or anxiety.

## Case Example: James's Tension Headache Control

James, a 45-year-old attorney, developed chronic tension headaches that seemed related to work stress. The headaches occurred daily and were affecting his concentration and work performance. Stress management techniques had provided minimal relief, and he wanted to avoid daily medication use.

His physician recommended biofeedback training to help him learn to control the muscle tension that contributed to his headaches. James was intrigued by the technological approach and appreciated the objective feedback about his physiological responses.

The biofeedback sessions began with EMG monitoring of his forehead and neck muscles. James could see his muscle tension levels displayed on a computer screen in real-time. He was surprised to discover how tense these muscles were even when he felt relatively relaxed.

The training taught James various relaxation techniques while he watched his muscle tension levels on the screen. He learned to breathe diaphragmatically, use progressive muscle relaxation, and employ mental imagery to reduce muscle tension. The immediate feedback helped him identify which techniques worked best for him.

James also learned to recognize early signs of increasing muscle tension throughout his day. He could catch tension building before it developed into a full headache and use his relaxation techniques to prevent the pain from escalating.

After 12 weeks of biofeedback training, James's headache frequency had decreased by 80%. He felt confident in his ability to manage stress and tension before they triggered headaches. The training provided him with practical skills that he could use independently.

**Breathing Techniques**

Breathing techniques represent one of the most accessible and effective mind-body approaches to pain management. These practices work by activating the parasympathetic nervous system, reducing stress hormones, and promoting relaxation responses that can significantly reduce pain intensity.

Research published in PubMed Central has documented the effectiveness of breathing techniques for various pain conditions (48, 49, 50, 51, 52, 53, 54, 55). The Cleveland Clinic and other major medical centers now recommend specific breathing exercises as part of pain management protocols.

Controlled breathing affects pain through multiple mechanisms. Slow, deep breathing activates the vagus nerve, which triggers the relaxation response. This physiological change reduces stress hormones that can amplify pain while promoting the release of endorphins that provide natural pain relief.

**Diaphragmatic Breathing for Pain Relief**

Diaphragmatic breathing, also called belly breathing, involves breathing deeply into the lower lungs using the diaphragm muscle.

This technique contrasts with shallow chest breathing that often accompanies stress and pain.

The practice involves placing one hand on the chest and another on the abdomen. During proper diaphragmatic breathing, the hand on the abdomen should rise and fall while the hand on the chest remains relatively still. This technique ensures that the diaphragm is doing the work of breathing rather than accessory muscles.

Regular practice of diaphragmatic breathing can reduce baseline stress levels and improve pain tolerance. The technique can also be used during pain flares to help manage acute increases in pain intensity.

### Case Example: Maria's Breathing Breakthrough

Maria, a 41-year-old social worker, developed chronic pain following a car accident. Her pain was accompanied by anxiety and panic attacks that seemed to make her pain worse. She found herself breathing shallowly and feeling constantly tense.

Her physical therapist taught Maria diaphragmatic breathing techniques as part of her pain management program. Initially, Maria struggled with the practice, finding it difficult to breathe deeply when she was in pain. The therapist assured her that this was normal and that skill would develop with practice.

Maria began practicing diaphragmatic breathing for five minutes twice daily. She gradually increased the duration as her skill improved. The practice helped her feel more relaxed and in control of her body's responses to pain.

During pain flares, Maria used breathing techniques to prevent panic and maintain calm. She discovered that focusing on her breath helped redirect her attention away from pain while promoting relaxation. This approach helped her manage flares more effectively without always relying on medication.

After several months of regular practice, Maria reported significant improvements in both pain intensity and anxiety levels. She felt more equipped to handle her chronic pain and had developed confidence in her ability to influence her pain experience through breathing.

## Advanced Breathing Techniques

Box breathing involves inhaling for four counts, holding for four counts, exhaling for four counts, and holding empty for four counts. This technique helps regulate the nervous system and can be particularly effective during stressful situations.

4-7-8 breathing involves inhaling for four counts, holding for seven counts, and exhaling for eight counts. This technique can be very effective for promoting relaxation and sleep, making it useful for people whose pain interferes with rest.

Coherent breathing involves maintaining a steady rhythm of five breaths per minute. This rate optimizes heart rate variability and can help synchronize various physiological systems for maximum relaxation benefit.

## Integration and Practice

The mind-body approaches described in this chapter work best when practiced regularly and integrated into daily life. These techniques require consistent practice to develop skill and achieve maximum benefit. The key is finding approaches that resonate with your preferences and lifestyle.

Many people benefit from combining multiple techniques. For example, someone might use CBT-P to address unhelpful thought patterns, practice mindfulness during daily activities, and use breathing techniques during pain flares. This combination approach can provide comprehensive mental training for pain management.

The skills learned through these approaches become more powerful with practice. Initial benefits may be modest, but continued practice typically leads to increasingly significant improvements in pain management and quality of life.

## Mental Training Foundations

The mind-body approaches to pain management represent scientifically validated treatments that can provide significant relief for chronic pain conditions. These techniques work by changing how your brain processes pain signals, reducing the emotional and cognitive factors that amplify suffering.

The key to success with these approaches is understanding that they require active participation and regular practice. Unlike taking medication, these techniques demand engagement and commitment. However, the skills you develop become lasting tools that can serve you throughout your life.

The next chapter will explore how lifestyle factors, particularly nutrition and diet, can influence pain levels and recovery. These foundational elements work synergistically with the mind-body approaches to create a comprehensive approach to pain management.

**Core Mind-Body Strategies:**

- CBT-P provides structured training to change pain-related thoughts and behaviors

- MBSR offers an eight-week program for developing mindfulness skills that transform your relationship with pain

- Clinical hypnotherapy accesses altered states of consciousness to modify pain perception

- Biofeedback training teaches conscious control over physiological processes that influence pain

- Breathing techniques offer accessible tools for activating relaxation responses and reducing pain intensity

- Regular practice and integration of multiple approaches optimize mind-body pain management benefits

# Chapter 8: The Anti-Inflammatory Lifestyle

Your daily choices create an internal environment that either promotes healing or perpetuates inflammation. This isn't about perfection or dramatic lifestyle overhauls - it's about understanding how food, sleep, stress, and hydration directly influence your pain levels and making informed decisions that support your recovery.

The connection between lifestyle and pain runs deeper than most people realize. Chronic inflammation provides the biological foundation for many pain conditions, and your daily habits can either fuel this inflammatory fire or help extinguish it. The encouraging news is that relatively modest changes can produce meaningful improvements in pain levels and quality of life.

### Food as Medicine

The Mediterranean diet has emerged as one of the most effective dietary approaches for reducing inflammation and managing pain. Research published by the Arthritis Foundation demonstrates that this eating pattern can significantly reduce inflammatory markers while improving pain outcomes across various conditions (56, 57, 58).

The Mediterranean diet isn't actually a diet in the traditional sense - it's a way of eating based on the traditional foods of countries bordering the Mediterranean Sea. This approach emphasizes whole foods, healthy fats, and anti-inflammatory compounds while limiting processed foods and refined sugars.

### Understanding Inflammatory vs. Anti-Inflammatory Foods

Foods can be broadly categorized based on their inflammatory potential. Pro-inflammatory foods tend to increase inflammatory markers in the blood and may worsen pain conditions. These include processed foods, refined sugars, trans fats, and excessive omega-6 fatty acids found in many vegetable oils.

Anti-inflammatory foods contain compounds that actively reduce inflammation in the body. These include fatty fish rich in omega-3 fatty acids, colorful fruits and vegetables high in antioxidants, nuts and seeds, and whole grains. The key is shifting the balance toward anti-inflammatory foods while reducing inflammatory ones.

The timing and combination of foods also matters. Eating anti-inflammatory foods together can enhance their benefits, while combining pro-inflammatory foods can amplify their negative effects. Understanding these interactions helps optimize your dietary approach for pain management.

### Case Example: Margaret's Dietary Transformation

Margaret, a 58-year-old office manager, had struggled with rheumatoid arthritis for over a decade. Despite medication, her joint pain and stiffness significantly limited her daily activities. She often felt exhausted and noticed that her pain seemed to fluctuate without clear patterns.

Her rheumatologist suggested that dietary changes might help reduce inflammation and improve her symptoms. Margaret was initially skeptical, having tried various diets without success. However, she agreed to work with a registered dietitian who specialized in inflammatory conditions.

The dietitian helped Margaret transition to a Mediterranean-style eating pattern. Instead of drastically eliminating foods, they focused on gradually adding anti-inflammatory options. Margaret began including fatty fish like salmon and sardines twice weekly, increased her vegetable intake, and switched to olive oil for cooking.

Margaret also learned to identify foods that seemed to trigger her symptoms. She discovered that processed foods and excess sugar consistently worsened her joint pain and fatigue. By tracking her food intake and symptoms, she could identify specific trigger foods.

The changes weren't immediate, but after six weeks, Margaret noticed improvements in her energy levels and joint stiffness. Her morning stiffness decreased from two hours to thirty minutes, and she felt less fatigued throughout the day. Lab tests showed reduced inflammatory markers.

After six months of following the Mediterranean diet, Margaret's pain levels had decreased by 40%. She was able to reduce one of her medications while maintaining better symptom control. Her case demonstrates how dietary changes can complement medical treatment for inflammatory conditions.

## Key Components of Anti-Inflammatory Eating

Omega-3 fatty acids represent one of the most powerful anti-inflammatory nutrients. Found in fatty fish, walnuts, flaxseeds, and chia seeds, these fats help produce compounds that actively resolve inflammation. The goal is to consume fatty fish at least twice weekly or consider supplementation if dietary intake is insufficient.

Antioxidants protect cells from inflammatory damage caused by free radicals. Colorful fruits and vegetables provide the widest range of antioxidants. The more colorful your plate, the more diverse your antioxidant intake. Berries, leafy greens, and brightly colored vegetables should feature prominently in anti-inflammatory eating.

Polyphenols are plant compounds that have potent anti-inflammatory effects. Found in foods like green tea, dark chocolate, red wine (in moderation), and colorful fruits, these compounds can help reduce inflammatory markers and may provide direct pain relief.

Fiber supports the beneficial bacteria in your gut, which play a crucial role in regulating inflammation throughout the body. Whole grains, legumes, fruits, and vegetables provide both soluble and insoluble fiber that supports gut health and reduces systemic inflammation.

## Case Example: Tom's Gut Health Journey

Tom, a 45-year-old construction worker, developed chronic low back pain that wasn't responding well to traditional treatments. He also struggled with digestive issues and noticed that his pain seemed worse after certain meals. His physician suggested that gut health might be contributing to his inflammation and pain.

Tom began working with a functional medicine practitioner who emphasized the connection between gut health and systemic inflammation. The treatment plan focused on healing his digestive system while reducing inflammatory foods.

Tom eliminated processed foods, refined sugars, and foods he suspected might be triggers. He increased his intake of fermented foods like yogurt and sauerkraut to support beneficial gut bacteria. He also added more fiber-rich foods to promote healthy digestion.

The practitioner recommended specific supplements to support gut healing, including probiotics and omega-3 fatty acids. Tom also learned stress management techniques, as chronic stress was contributing to his digestive problems.

After two months, Tom noticed significant improvements in both his digestive symptoms and back pain. His energy levels increased, and he felt less inflammation throughout his body. The connection between his gut health and pain became clear as both improved together.

Tom's case illustrates how addressing underlying gut health issues can provide unexpected benefits for pain management. The anti-inflammatory approach helped him address multiple health concerns simultaneously.

**Elimination Diets for Pain Management**

Elimination diets can help identify specific foods that trigger inflammation and worsen pain. This systematic approach involves removing potential trigger foods for a specific period, then reintroducing them one at a time to identify individual sensitivities.

The process requires patience and careful tracking, but it can provide valuable information about foods that specifically affect your pain levels. Common trigger foods include dairy products, gluten-containing grains, nightshade vegetables, and certain food additives.

**The Elimination Diet Process**

The elimination phase typically lasts 3-4 weeks and involves removing all potential trigger foods from your diet. This period allows inflammation to decrease and symptoms to stabilize. During this phase, you focus on eating whole, unprocessed foods that are unlikely to cause reactions.

The reintroduction phase involves adding back one food group at a time while carefully monitoring symptoms. Each food group is tested for 3-4 days before adding the next one. This systematic approach helps identify specific foods that trigger symptoms.

Documentation is crucial throughout the process. You'll track what you eat, how you feel, and any changes in pain levels. This information helps identify patterns and specific trigger foods.

## Case Example: Jennifer's Food Detective Work

Jennifer, a 34-year-old teacher, experienced chronic headaches and joint pain that seemed unrelated to any specific injury or condition. Her symptoms varied significantly from day to day, making it difficult to identify patterns. Her physician suggested that food sensitivities might be contributing to her symptoms.

Jennifer worked with a registered dietitian to design an elimination diet protocol. She removed dairy, gluten, eggs, soy, and nightshade vegetables from her diet for four weeks. The initial adjustment was challenging, but she noticed gradual improvements in her symptoms.

During the elimination phase, Jennifer's headaches decreased from daily to twice weekly. Her joint pain also improved, and she felt less overall inflammation. These improvements motivated her to continue with the reintroduction phase.

The reintroduction phase revealed that dairy products were a significant trigger for Jennifer's headaches. When she reintroduced dairy after four weeks without it, her headaches returned within 24 hours. Gluten also seemed to worsen her joint pain, though the effect was less dramatic.

Jennifer modified her diet to avoid dairy and reduce gluten intake. She found suitable alternatives that allowed her to maintain a varied, enjoyable diet while avoiding trigger foods. Her headaches decreased by 80%, and her joint pain improved significantly.

## Hydration and Pain Management

Proper hydration plays a crucial but often overlooked role in pain management. Dehydration can increase pain sensitivity, worsen inflammation, and impair the body's natural healing processes. Understanding the connection between hydration and pain can help you optimize this simple but powerful tool.

Water is essential for numerous physiological processes that affect pain. It helps transport nutrients to tissues, remove waste products, and maintain proper blood flow. Dehydration can disrupt these processes, potentially increasing pain sensitivity and slowing healing.

## The Hydration-Pain Connection

Dehydration affects pain through multiple mechanisms. When you're dehydrated, your blood becomes more concentrated, making it harder for your cardiovascular system to deliver oxygen and nutrients to tissues. This can increase inflammation and pain sensitivity.

Dehydration also affects the nervous system's ability to regulate pain signals. Proper hydration is necessary for optimal nerve function, and even mild dehydration can affect pain processing. This may explain why some people notice increased pain during hot weather or after intense exercise.

Joint health depends on proper hydration because cartilage is composed largely of water. Dehydration can affect joint lubrication and increase stiffness, particularly in people with arthritis or other joint conditions.

## Optimizing Hydration for Pain Relief

The traditional recommendation of eight glasses of water daily provides a starting point, but individual needs vary based on activity level, climate, and overall health. A better approach is to monitor your hydration status and adjust intake accordingly.

Urine color provides a simple indicator of hydration status. Pale yellow indicates good hydration, while dark yellow suggests dehydration. Very clear urine might indicate overhydration, which can also cause problems.

The timing of fluid intake matters for pain management. Drinking water consistently throughout the day maintains steady hydration levels. Drinking large amounts infrequently can stress the kidneys and doesn't provide optimal hydration.

## Sleep Optimization for Pain Relief

The relationship between sleep and pain is bidirectional and powerful. Poor sleep increases pain sensitivity, while pain can disrupt sleep quality, creating a vicious cycle that perpetuates chronic pain conditions. Breaking this cycle requires addressing both sleep quality and pain management simultaneously.

Sleep serves crucial functions for pain management and healing. During deep sleep, the body releases growth hormone, which promotes tissue repair and reduces inflammation. Sleep also helps regulate pain-processing chemicals in the brain.

## Understanding Sleep-Pain Interactions

Sleep deprivation directly increases pain sensitivity through measurable changes in brain function. Even one night of poor sleep can increase pain sensitivity by 15-20%. Chronic sleep problems can lead to persistent increases in pain intensity.

Sleep disorders are common in people with chronic pain conditions. Sleep apnea, restless leg syndrome, and other disorders can disrupt sleep quality and worsen pain. Addressing these underlying sleep disorders often improves pain management.

The timing of sleep matters for pain management. Consistent sleep and wake times help regulate circadian rhythms, which affect pain sensitivity. Irregular sleep schedules can disrupt these natural rhythms and increase pain.

## Sleep Hygiene for Pain Management

Creating an optimal sleep environment supports both sleep quality and pain management. The bedroom should be cool, dark, and quiet. Comfortable bedding and mattresses are particularly important for people with pain conditions.

Evening routines can help signal to your body that it's time to sleep. This might include dimming lights, avoiding screens, and engaging in relaxing activities. Consistency in these routines helps regulate sleep-wake cycles.

Managing pain that interferes with sleep requires specific strategies. This might include timing pain medications to provide relief during sleep hours, using heat or cold therapy before bed, or practicing relaxation techniques to manage pain-related anxiety.

## Stress Management for Pain Control

Chronic stress creates a biological environment that promotes inflammation and increases pain sensitivity. Stress hormones like cortisol can amplify pain signals while suppressing the body's natural healing processes. Effective stress management is therefore essential for optimal pain control.

The connection between stress and pain isn't just psychological - it's measurable at the cellular level. Chronic stress triggers inflammatory pathways that can worsen pain conditions and slow healing. Managing stress can therefore provide direct benefits for pain management.

## Stress-Pain Physiology

Stress activates the hypothalamic-pituitary-adrenal (HPA) axis, leading to the release of stress hormones. These hormones can increase inflammation, suppress immune function, and increase pain sensitivity. Chronic activation of this system can contribute to persistent pain conditions.

Stress also affects sleep quality, which as discussed above, directly impacts pain sensitivity. The combination of stress and poor sleep creates a particularly challenging situation for pain management.

Muscle tension often accompanies stress and can directly contribute to pain conditions. Stress-related muscle tension can worsen headaches, back pain, and other musculoskeletal conditions.

### Practical Stress Management Techniques

Progressive muscle relaxation involves systematically tensing and releasing muscle groups throughout the body. This technique can help reduce stress-related muscle tension while promoting overall relaxation.

Mindfulness-based stress reduction, discussed in the previous chapter, provides structured training in managing stress responses. Regular mindfulness practice can help you respond to stressors more effectively and reduce their impact on pain.

Time management and lifestyle modifications can help reduce chronic stress. This might involve setting boundaries, delegating responsibilities, or making changes to reduce daily stressors that contribute to pain.

### Lifestyle Integration Strategies

Creating an anti-inflammatory lifestyle requires integrating multiple approaches rather than focusing on any single intervention. The key is making sustainable changes that you can maintain long-term rather than attempting dramatic overhauls that are difficult to sustain.

Start with small, manageable changes that build on each other. For example, you might begin by adding one anti-inflammatory food to your daily diet, then gradually expand to include more beneficial foods while reducing inflammatory ones.

The timing of lifestyle changes can affect their success. Some people do better making gradual changes, while others prefer more dramatic shifts. The key is finding an approach that fits your personality and circumstances.

**Holistic Health Foundations**

The anti-inflammatory lifestyle approach recognizes that pain management extends far beyond medical treatments to include the daily choices that create your internal environment. Food, sleep, stress, and hydration all directly influence pain levels and recovery potential.

The power of lifestyle approaches lies in their cumulative effect. Small improvements in multiple areas can produce significant overall benefits for pain management and quality of life. The key is consistency and patience as these changes take time to produce their full benefits.

The next chapter will explore specific supplements and natural remedies that can complement lifestyle approaches. These targeted interventions can provide additional support for pain management when used appropriately as part of a comprehensive approach.

**Lifestyle Modification Principles:**

- Mediterranean-style eating patterns provide powerful anti-inflammatory benefits for pain management

- Elimination diets can identify specific food triggers that worsen pain and inflammation

- Proper hydration supports optimal pain processing and tissue healing

- Quality sleep is essential for pain regulation and recovery

- Effective stress management reduces inflammation and pain sensitivity

- Sustainable lifestyle changes require gradual implementation and long-term commitment

# Chapter 9: Evidence-Based Supplements and Natural Remedies

The supplement industry generates billions of dollars annually, yet many products lack scientific support for their claimed benefits. This chapter cuts through the marketing hype to focus on natural remedies with solid research backing their use for pain management. The goal isn't to replace conventional treatments but to identify evidence-based supplements that can enhance your pain management strategy.

Understanding which supplements actually work - and which are merely expensive placebos - empowers you to make informed decisions about incorporating these products into your pain management plan. The key lies in focusing on supplements with substantial research support while maintaining realistic expectations about their benefits.

## The Big Three Evidence-Based Supplements

Three supplements stand out for their robust research support and clinical effectiveness in pain management: turmeric (curcumin), omega-3 fatty acids, and vitamin D. These compounds have been extensively studied and show consistent benefits across multiple pain conditions.

## Turmeric and Curcumin

Turmeric contains curcumin, a compound with powerful anti-inflammatory properties that have been extensively researched. Studies published in major medical journals have documented curcumin's effectiveness for various pain conditions, with benefits comparable to some prescription medications (59, 60, 61).

Curcumin works through multiple mechanisms to reduce inflammation and pain. It inhibits several inflammatory pathways while promoting the resolution of inflammation. This dual action makes it particularly effective for conditions involving chronic inflammation.

The challenge with curcumin lies in its poor bioavailability - the body doesn't absorb it well in its natural form. However, newer formulations combine curcumin with compounds like piperine (from black pepper) or phospholipids to enhance absorption significantly.

**Case Example: Patricia's Arthritis Success**

Patricia, a 64-year-old retired nurse, had struggled with osteoarthritis in her knees for several years. The pain was limiting her ability to walk and garden, activities she had always enjoyed. Traditional anti-inflammatory medications provided some relief but caused stomach upset that made them difficult to tolerate.

Her physician suggested trying a high-quality curcumin supplement as a natural alternative. Patricia was skeptical about supplements but agreed to try curcumin for three months to see if it would help her symptoms.

Patricia chose a curcumin supplement that included piperine to enhance absorption. She took 500mg twice daily with meals, as recommended by her physician. She noticed gradual improvements in her knee pain and stiffness over the first month.

After three months of consistent use, Patricia's knee pain had decreased by approximately 50%. She was able to walk longer distances and resume gardening with minimal discomfort. Her physician confirmed that her inflammatory markers had decreased significantly.

Patricia has continued taking curcumin for over a year with sustained benefits. She's been able to reduce her use of over-the-counter pain medications while maintaining better pain control. Her case demonstrates how curcumin can provide meaningful relief for inflammatory pain conditions.

## Omega-3 Fatty Acids

Omega-3 fatty acids, particularly EPA and DHA found in fish oil, have extensive research support for their anti-inflammatory and pain-reducing effects. These essential fatty acids help produce compounds that actively resolve inflammation rather than simply blocking it.

The standard American diet tends to be high in omega-6 fatty acids and low in omega-3s, creating an inflammatory imbalance. Supplementing with omega-3s can help restore this balance and reduce systemic inflammation.

Research supports omega-3 supplementation for various pain conditions, including rheumatoid arthritis, back pain, and general inflammatory conditions. The anti-inflammatory effects typically require several weeks of consistent supplementation to become apparent.

## Vitamin D for Pain Management

Vitamin D deficiency is common and has been linked to increased pain sensitivity and various pain conditions. This nutrient functions more like a hormone than a traditional vitamin, affecting immune function and inflammation regulation.

Research shows that people with chronic pain conditions often have low vitamin D levels. Correcting deficiency through supplementation can provide significant pain relief for some individuals, particularly those with musculoskeletal pain.

The connection between vitamin D and pain involves multiple mechanisms. Vitamin D receptors are found throughout the nervous system, and adequate levels are necessary for optimal nerve function. Deficiency can increase pain sensitivity and worsen inflammatory conditions.

## Case Example: Robert's Vitamin D Discovery

Robert, a 52-year-old accountant, had experienced chronic muscle pain and fatigue for over two years. Despite extensive medical evaluation, no specific cause was identified. His symptoms were affecting his work performance and quality of life.

During routine blood work, Robert's physician discovered that his vitamin D level was severely deficient at 12 ng/mL (normal is above 30 ng/mL). Given the connection between vitamin D deficiency and pain, his physician recommended aggressive supplementation.

Robert began taking 4,000 IU of vitamin D3 daily, along with magnesium to support absorption. His physician monitored his blood levels to ensure they reached optimal ranges. Robert also increased his sun exposure when possible.

After two months of supplementation, Robert noticed significant improvements in his muscle pain and energy levels. His sleep quality improved, and he felt less stiff and sore throughout the day. Follow-up blood work showed his vitamin D level had increased to 45 ng/mL.

Robert's case illustrates how correcting vitamin D deficiency can provide dramatic pain relief for some individuals. The supplement was simple and inexpensive, yet it provided benefits that multiple other treatments hadn't achieved.

### Joint Support Supplements

Glucosamine and chondroitin represent the most studied supplements for joint pain, though research results have been mixed. These compounds are natural components of cartilage and theoretically should support joint health, but clinical trials have shown variable results.

### Glucosamine and Chondroitin Research

Multiple large-scale studies have examined glucosamine and chondroitin for osteoarthritis. While some studies show modest benefits, others find no significant effects. The variability in results may be due to differences in supplement quality, dosing, and study populations (62, 63, 64, 65, 66, 67, 68, 69, 70).

Harvard Health has published analysis suggesting that glucosamine and chondroitin may provide modest benefits for some people with osteoarthritis, particularly those with moderate to severe symptoms (71). However, the effects are generally smaller than those seen with prescription medications.

The supplements appear to be most effective for people with mild to moderate osteoarthritis. They may help slow cartilage breakdown and provide modest pain relief, but they're unlikely to provide dramatic improvements in severe cases.

### Case Example: Susan's Mixed Results

Susan, a 61-year-old teacher, developed osteoarthritis in her hands that was affecting her ability to write and perform daily tasks. She preferred to avoid prescription medications if possible and wanted to try natural approaches first.

Susan began taking glucosamine sulfate and chondroitin sulfate as recommended by her pharmacist. She took the supplements consistently for six months, following the dosing instructions carefully.

Initially, Susan didn't notice any significant changes in her symptoms. However, after about three months, she began to feel that her joints were slightly less stiff in the morning. The improvement was subtle but consistent.

After six months of supplementation, Susan felt that her joint pain had decreased by about 20-30%. While this wasn't dramatic relief, it was enough to improve her daily function and delay the need for prescription medications.

Susan's case illustrates the typical experience with glucosamine and chondroitin - modest benefits that may be worthwhile for some people, but not the dramatic improvements that marketing claims might suggest.

## Other Joint Support Compounds

Methylsulfonylmethane (MSM) is another popular joint supplement with limited research support. Some studies suggest it may provide modest anti-inflammatory effects, but the evidence is not as robust as for other supplements.

Hyaluronic acid supplements are marketed for joint health, but oral supplements are poorly absorbed and unlikely to reach joint tissues in meaningful concentrations. Topical applications may be more effective for localized joint pain.

Boswellia serrata extract has shown promise in some studies for inflammatory joint conditions. This herbal remedy appears to have anti-inflammatory effects, though more research is needed to confirm its effectiveness.

## Nerve Support Supplements

Neuropathic pain conditions often respond to specific nutrients that support nerve function and reduce inflammation in the nervous system. These supplements can be particularly helpful for people with diabetic neuropathy, postherpetic neuralgia, and other nerve-related pain conditions.

## B Vitamins for Nerve Health

B vitamins, particularly B1 (thiamine), B6 (pyridoxine), and B12 (cobalamin), are essential for proper nerve function. Deficiencies in these vitamins can contribute to neuropathic pain, and supplementation may provide relief for some individuals.

B12 deficiency is particularly common in older adults and vegetarians. This deficiency can cause numbness, tingling, and pain that may be mistaken for other conditions. Correcting B12 deficiency can provide significant relief for affected individuals.

B6 supplementation may help with certain types of nerve pain, but excessive doses can actually cause nerve damage. The key is using appropriate doses under professional guidance.

### Alpha-Lipoic Acid

Alpha-lipoic acid is a powerful antioxidant that has shown particular promise for diabetic neuropathy. This compound can help protect nerve cells from damage while potentially improving nerve function.

Research suggests that alpha-lipoic acid may help reduce pain and improve nerve function in people with diabetic neuropathy. The effects appear to be dose-dependent, with higher doses (600-1800mg daily) showing better results.

### Magnesium for Nerve Function

Magnesium plays crucial roles in nerve function and muscle relaxation. Deficiency is common and can contribute to muscle cramps, tension, and nerve pain. Supplementation may help with certain types of pain, particularly muscle-related conditions.

Magnesium can also help with sleep quality, which is important for pain management. Different forms of magnesium have different absorption rates and effects, so choosing the right form is important.

### Supplement Quality and Safety

The supplement industry is poorly regulated, and product quality varies dramatically between manufacturers. Understanding how to choose high-quality supplements is crucial for both safety and effectiveness.

### Third-Party Testing

Look for supplements that have been tested by independent third parties for purity and potency. Organizations like USP (United States Pharmacopeia), NSF International, and ConsumerLab provide testing services that verify supplement quality.

Third-party testing ensures that supplements contain what their labels claim and are free from contaminants. This is particularly important for supplements manufactured overseas or by smaller companies.

## Absorption and Bioavailability

The form of a supplement affects how well your body can absorb and use it. For example, magnesium glycinate is better absorbed than magnesium oxide. Similarly, curcumin with piperine is better absorbed than curcumin alone.

Some supplements work better when taken with food, while others are better absorbed on an empty stomach. Understanding these factors can help you optimize supplement effectiveness.

## Standardization

Look for supplements that are standardized to specific active compounds. For example, a curcumin supplement should specify the percentage of curcuminoids it contains. This ensures consistent potency between batches.

## Drug-Supplement Interactions

Supplements can interact with prescription medications, potentially affecting their effectiveness or causing adverse reactions. Always inform your healthcare providers about all supplements you're taking.

## Common Interactions

Fish oil supplements can increase bleeding risk when combined with blood-thinning medications like warfarin. Turmeric can have similar effects and may also interact with diabetes medications.

Some supplements can affect liver enzymes that metabolize medications, potentially altering drug levels in the body. This is particularly important for people taking medications with narrow therapeutic windows.

## Timing Considerations

Some supplements can interfere with medication absorption if taken at the same time. For example, calcium and magnesium can reduce the absorption of certain antibiotics. Timing doses several hours apart can prevent these interactions.

## Professional Guidance

While many supplements are available over-the-counter, professional guidance can help you choose appropriate products and avoid potential problems. Healthcare providers can help you navigate the complex world of supplements safely and effectively.

## When to Consult Professionals

Consider consulting with a healthcare provider before starting supplements if you have chronic health conditions, take prescription medications, or have had previous adverse reactions to supplements.

Pharmacists can provide valuable advice about supplement-drug interactions and help you choose high-quality products. Many pharmacists have specialized training in natural products and can provide evidence-based recommendations.

## Monitoring and Adjustment

Some supplements require monitoring to ensure safety and effectiveness. For example, high-dose vitamin D supplementation requires periodic blood tests to prevent toxicity. Iron supplements need monitoring to prevent overload.

Regular evaluation of supplement effectiveness is important. If a supplement isn't providing benefits after an appropriate trial period, it may be time to discontinue it or try alternatives.

## Evidence-Based Approach

The key to successful supplement use lies in focusing on products with solid research support while maintaining realistic expectations. Supplements work best as part of a comprehensive pain management plan that includes lifestyle modifications and appropriate medical care.

Quality matters significantly in supplement effectiveness. Investing in high-quality products from reputable manufacturers is more likely to provide benefits than using cheaper alternatives of questionable quality.

The next chapter will explore condition-specific protocols that integrate supplements with other evidence-based treatments. These targeted approaches can help you develop a comprehensive plan tailored to your specific pain condition.

**Natural Remedy Conclusions**

Evidence-based supplements can provide meaningful support for pain management when used appropriately. The key is focusing on products with solid research support while avoiding the countless supplements that lack scientific backing.

Success with supplements requires patience, as most natural remedies take weeks or months to show their full effects. They work best as part of a comprehensive approach that includes appropriate lifestyle modifications and medical care when needed.

The supplement industry will continue to evolve, with new products and formulations constantly emerging. Staying informed about current research helps you make educated decisions about which supplements might benefit your specific situation.

**Research-Supported Supplement Strategies:**

- Turmeric, omega-3 fatty acids, and vitamin D have the strongest research support for pain management

- Glucosamine and chondroitin may provide modest benefits for joint pain but effects are generally limited

- B vitamins, alpha-lipoic acid, and magnesium can support nerve function and reduce neuropathic pain

- Supplement quality varies dramatically, making third-party testing and reputable manufacturers essential

- Drug-supplement interactions require professional guidance to avoid adverse effects

- Evidence-based selection and realistic expectations optimize supplement benefits for pain management

# Chapter 10: Back and Neck Pain Solutions

Nearly 80% of adults will experience back pain at some point in their lives, making it one of the most common reasons people seek medical care. Yet despite its prevalence, back and neck pain often becomes a source of frustration for both patients and healthcare providers. The good news is that evidence-based approaches can provide meaningful relief for most people - the key lies in understanding which treatments actually work and implementing them correctly.

The spine is a marvel of engineering, providing both stability and mobility while protecting the delicate spinal cord. When this system breaks down, the resulting pain can be debilitating. However, modern pain science has revealed that most spinal pain is not caused by serious structural problems but rather by muscle tension, inflammation, and changes in how the nervous system processes pain signals.

**Lower Back Pain and the Evidence-Based Protocol**

The American College of Physicians has developed clear, evidence-based guidelines for treating low back pain that represent a significant departure from traditional approaches (72, 73, 74, 75, 76). These guidelines emphasize non-drug treatments as first-line therapy, reserving medications for specific situations where they've proven beneficial.

The protocol begins with education and reassurance. Most episodes of acute low back pain resolve on their own within a few weeks, and the vast majority of people can expect to return to normal activities. This message is crucial because fear and anxiety about back pain often worsen the condition and delay recovery.

Heat therapy emerges as one of the most effective immediate treatments for acute low back pain. Applied for 15-20 minutes several times daily, heat can reduce muscle tension and provide meaningful pain relief. The mechanism involves increasing blood flow to the area while activating sensory nerve fibers that can block pain signals.

## Case Example: Maria's Acute Back Pain Recovery

Maria, a 38-year-old teacher, developed severe low back pain after lifting boxes while setting up her classroom. The pain was sharp and limiting, making it difficult to stand or walk. She was concerned about potential disc damage and worried about missing work during the first week of school.

Her physician assessed her condition and found no red flag symptoms suggesting serious pathology. Following the ACP guidelines, he recommended against immediate imaging and instead focused on evidence-based conservative treatment. He reassured Maria that her pain was likely due to muscle strain and would improve with appropriate care.

The treatment plan included heat therapy, gentle movement, and a gradual return to normal activities. Maria applied heat for 20 minutes three times daily, which provided immediate relief from muscle tension. She was encouraged to remain active within her pain tolerance rather than staying in bed.

Maria also received education about pain mechanisms and the importance of movement for recovery. She learned that bed rest could actually delay healing and that gradual activity was beneficial. This understanding helped reduce her anxiety about movement and motivated her to stay active.

Within one week, Maria's pain had decreased by 60%. She was able to return to teaching with some modifications, using proper lifting techniques and taking breaks to apply heat when needed. Her case demonstrates how following evidence-based guidelines can lead to rapid improvement in acute back pain.

## Movement as Medicine for Back Pain

The evidence strongly supports early mobilization and exercise for back pain recovery. Bed rest, once considered essential for back pain treatment, is now known to delay recovery and can actually worsen pain in many cases. The key is finding the right balance between rest and activity.

Gentle stretching and strengthening exercises should begin as soon as possible after the acute phase. These exercises help maintain flexibility, reduce muscle tension, and prevent deconditioning. The specific exercises should be tailored to individual needs and pain levels.

Walking represents one of the best exercises for back pain recovery. It's low-impact, accessible, and helps maintain overall fitness while promoting healing. Starting with short walks and gradually increasing duration and intensity provides a structured approach to recovery.

**Manual Therapy Integration**

The ACP guidelines support the use of spinal manipulation and massage therapy for acute low back pain. These treatments can provide short-term pain relief and may help people return to normal activities more quickly. However, they work best when combined with exercise and education rather than used as standalone treatments.

Massage therapy can help reduce muscle tension and promote relaxation, which are often beneficial for back pain recovery. The treatment should focus on the affected muscles and surrounding areas, using techniques that promote circulation and reduce inflammation.

Spinal manipulation by qualified practitioners can provide immediate pain relief for some people with acute back pain. The treatment involves applying controlled force to specific spinal joints to improve mobility and reduce pain. Success depends on proper patient selection and skilled application.

**Neck Pain and Whiplash Recovery**

Neck pain affects millions of Americans annually, with causes ranging from poor posture to motor vehicle accidents. Whiplash injuries, in particular, can lead to persistent pain and disability if not managed properly. The key to successful recovery lies in early intervention and appropriate treatment selection.

Whiplash occurs when the head is suddenly jerked forward and backward, causing strain to the neck muscles and ligaments. While many people recover completely within a few weeks, some develop chronic symptoms that can persist for months or years. Early, appropriate treatment can prevent this progression to chronicity.

**Case Example: David's Whiplash Recovery**

David, a 45-year-old accountant, was rear-ended at a traffic light, resulting in typical whiplash injuries. Initially, his neck pain was mild, but it worsened over the following days. He developed headaches, stiffness, and difficulty concentrating at work.

His physician diagnosed whiplash and recommended active treatment rather than immobilization. David was given a soft collar to use sparingly for comfort but was encouraged to maintain normal neck movements as much as possible. The goal was to prevent stiffness and muscle weakening.

The treatment plan included gentle neck exercises, heat therapy, and manual therapy. David performed range-of-motion exercises throughout the day, gradually increasing the extent of movement as his pain allowed. He applied heat for 15 minutes several times daily to reduce muscle tension.

David also received massage therapy twice weekly for the first month after his injury. The massage helped reduce muscle spasm and improved his range of motion. He was taught proper posture techniques and ergonomic adjustments for his workspace.

After six weeks of active treatment, David's symptoms had resolved almost completely. He returned to full work activities and resumed his normal exercise routine. His case illustrates how early, active treatment can prevent the development of chronic whiplash symptoms.

## Posture and Ergonomics for Neck Pain

Modern life creates numerous challenges for neck health, particularly for people who spend long hours working at computers. Poor posture, inadequate workspace setup, and repetitive motions can all contribute to neck pain and dysfunction. Addressing these factors is essential for both treatment and prevention.

Forward head posture, where the head juts forward from the shoulders, is extremely common and creates significant stress on the neck muscles. This posture increases the effective weight of the head that the neck muscles must support, leading to fatigue and pain.

Ergonomic workstation setup can significantly reduce neck strain. Monitor height should position the top of the screen at eye level, reducing the need to look up or down. Keyboard and mouse placement should allow the shoulders to remain relaxed while working.

## Sciatica Relief Through Targeted Approaches

Sciatica - pain that radiates from the low back down the leg - affects millions of Americans and can be one of the most debilitating forms of back pain. The condition occurs when the sciatic nerve becomes compressed or irritated, often due to a herniated disc or spinal stenosis.

The pain of sciatica is typically sharp, burning, or shooting, and it may be accompanied by numbness, tingling, or weakness in the leg. The intensity can range from mild discomfort to severe pain that makes walking or sitting nearly impossible.

## Case Example: Susan's Sciatica Success

Susan, a 52-year-old nurse, developed severe sciatica after a long shift of lifting patients. The pain started in her lower back but quickly spread down her right leg to her foot. She experienced numbness in her toes and weakness in her leg that made walking difficult.

Her physician performed a thorough evaluation and found evidence of nerve compression but no signs of serious complications requiring immediate surgery. The treatment plan focused on reducing inflammation and nerve irritation while promoting healing.

Susan began with anti-inflammatory medication and activity modification. She avoided positions and activities that worsened her symptoms while maintaining light activity as tolerated. She used ice therapy during the acute phase to reduce inflammation around the compressed nerve.

Physical therapy began once her acute symptoms improved. The program included specific exercises to reduce pressure on the sciatic nerve, strengthen supporting muscles, and improve flexibility. Susan learned techniques for proper lifting and body mechanics to prevent recurrence.

After eight weeks of conservative treatment, Susan's sciatica had resolved almost completely. She was able to return to work full-time with proper body mechanics and ergonomic modifications. Her case demonstrates how conservative treatment can effectively manage even severe sciatica.

**Understanding Nerve Pain vs. Muscle Pain**

Sciatica differs from typical back pain because it involves nerve irritation rather than just muscle strain. This distinction is important because nerve pain often requires different treatment approaches than muscle-related pain.

Nerve pain tends to be sharp, burning, or shooting, while muscle pain is typically aching or throbbing. Nerve pain may be accompanied by numbness, tingling, or weakness, while muscle pain usually doesn't cause these neurological symptoms.

The treatment approach for sciatica focuses on reducing nerve irritation and inflammation rather than just treating muscle tension. This may involve specific positions, exercises, and treatments that take pressure off the affected nerve.

## Posture and Ergonomics as Prevention

The old saying "an ounce of prevention is worth a pound of cure" is particularly relevant for spinal health. Many cases of back and neck pain can be prevented through proper posture, ergonomic workspaces, and healthy movement habits.

Modern lifestyles create numerous challenges for spinal health. Prolonged sitting, poor workstation setup, and repetitive motions all contribute to increased rates of back and neck pain. Addressing these factors proactively can prevent many problems from developing.

### Workplace Ergonomics

Proper workstation setup is crucial for people who spend long hours at computers. The monitor should be positioned at eye level to prevent neck strain, while the keyboard and mouse should allow the arms to remain relaxed at the sides.

Chair height should position the feet flat on the floor with the knees at approximately 90 degrees. The chair should provide adequate lumbar support to maintain the natural curve of the lower back. Armrests should support the arms without forcing the shoulders upward.

Taking regular breaks from sitting is essential for spinal health. The recommendation is to stand and move for at least two minutes every hour. This movement helps prevent muscle fatigue and maintains spinal flexibility.

### Daily Movement Habits

The way you move throughout the day significantly impacts spinal health. Proper lifting techniques, using leg muscles rather than back muscles, can prevent many injuries. The key is to keep the load close to the body while maintaining proper spinal alignment.

Sleeping position also affects spinal health. Side sleeping with a pillow between the knees helps maintain spinal alignment, while back sleeping may require a pillow under the knees. Stomach sleeping is generally discouraged as it can strain the neck and back.

Regular exercise is one of the most effective ways to prevent back and neck pain. Activities that strengthen the core muscles, maintain flexibility, and promote good posture can significantly reduce the risk of spinal problems.

## When to Seek Professional Help

While most episodes of back and neck pain resolve with conservative treatment, certain signs and symptoms require immediate medical attention. These "red flags" may indicate serious underlying conditions that need prompt evaluation and treatment.

## Red Flag Symptoms

Severe pain following trauma, such as a fall or motor vehicle accident, requires immediate evaluation to rule out fractures or other serious injuries. Any neurological symptoms, including weakness, numbness, or tingling in the arms or legs, should be evaluated promptly.

Bowel or bladder dysfunction in association with back pain can indicate cauda equina syndrome, a medical emergency that requires immediate surgical intervention. Fever accompanying back pain may suggest infection, which also requires urgent treatment.

Progressive neurological symptoms, such as increasing weakness or numbness, should be evaluated promptly even if they develop gradually. These symptoms may indicate nerve compression that could lead to permanent damage if not treated appropriately.

## When Conservative Treatment Isn't Enough

Most episodes of back and neck pain improve with conservative treatment within a few weeks. However, pain that persists beyond 6-8 weeks may require additional evaluation and treatment. This doesn't necessarily mean surgery is needed, but it does warrant reassessment.

Imaging studies like MRI or CT scans are typically reserved for cases where conservative treatment has failed or when red flag symptoms are present. These tests can identify specific structural problems that might require different treatment approaches.

Referral to specialists may be appropriate for complex cases or when conservative treatment hasn't provided adequate relief. Pain management specialists, orthopedic surgeons, and neurosurgeons all play roles in treating complex spinal conditions.

## The Path to Recovery

Back and neck pain can be frustrating and disabling, but the vast majority of people can expect to recover with appropriate treatment. The key is using evidence-based approaches that address the underlying causes of pain while promoting healing and preventing recurrence.

Success requires patience and persistence. Most spinal conditions improve gradually over weeks or months rather than days. Maintaining realistic expectations and staying committed to treatment recommendations are essential for optimal outcomes.

The next chapter will explore arthritis and joint pain management, conditions that often coexist with spinal problems and require similar multidisciplinary approaches for optimal management.

## Spinal Health Summary

Evidence-based treatment of back and neck pain has moved away from passive approaches toward active management that emphasizes movement, education, and gradual return to normal activities. The American College of Physicians guidelines provide a clear framework for effective treatment that can help most people recover from these common conditions.

Prevention remains the best strategy for spinal health. Proper ergonomics, regular exercise, and healthy movement habits can prevent many episodes of back and neck pain. When problems do occur, early intervention with appropriate treatment can prevent them from becoming chronic.

**Essential Spinal Care Strategies:**

- The ACP evidence-based protocol emphasizes non-drug treatments as first-line therapy for back pain

- Heat therapy and early mobilization are more effective than bed rest for acute back pain

- Whiplash recovery requires active treatment and proper ergonomics to prevent chronic symptoms

- Sciatica can often be managed conservatively with targeted exercises and activity modification

- Workplace ergonomics and proper posture are essential for preventing spinal problems

- Red flag symptoms require immediate medical evaluation to rule out serious conditions

# Chapter 11: Arthritis and Joint Pain Management

Arthritis affects more than 54 million Americans, making it one of the leading causes of disability in the United States. Yet many people accept joint pain as an inevitable part of aging, unaware that effective treatments can significantly reduce pain and improve function. The key lies in understanding that arthritis is not a single disease but rather a group of conditions requiring different approaches for optimal management.

The landscape of arthritis treatment has changed dramatically over the past decade. New medications, advanced understanding of inflammation, and evidence-based non-drug approaches have expanded treatment options significantly. Most importantly, early intervention can prevent or slow joint damage, making timely diagnosis and treatment crucial for long-term outcomes.

## Osteoarthritis and Evidence-Based Management

Osteoarthritis (OA) is the most common form of arthritis, affecting over 32 million Americans. This "wear and tear" arthritis involves the gradual breakdown of cartilage in joints, leading to pain, stiffness, and reduced function. The condition most commonly affects weight-bearing joints like the knees and hips, but it can occur in any joint.

The American College of Rheumatology and Arthritis Foundation have developed comprehensive guidelines for OA management that emphasize a multimodal approach combining non-drug and drug treatments (77). These guidelines represent a significant shift from purely symptom-focused care to comprehensive management that addresses function and quality of life.

## Understanding Osteoarthritis Progression

OA develops gradually over years or decades, making early intervention crucial for preventing progression. The condition involves more than just cartilage breakdown - it affects the entire joint, including bones, ligaments, and surrounding muscles. This understanding has led to treatment approaches that address all components of joint health.

The NCCIH has reviewed extensive research on complementary approaches to OA management, finding that several non-drug treatments can provide meaningful benefits (78). These approaches work best when combined with conventional treatments rather than used as replacements.

Risk factors for OA include age, obesity, previous joint injuries, and genetic predisposition. While some factors like age and genetics cannot be changed, others like weight and activity level can be modified to reduce disease progression and improve symptoms.

**Case Example: Robert's Knee Osteoarthritis Management**

Robert, a 62-year-old retired teacher, developed knee osteoarthritis that gradually worsened over several years. Initially, he experienced stiffness in the morning and pain after prolonged walking. Over time, the pain became more constant and began limiting his daily activities.

His rheumatologist diagnosed moderate osteoarthritis based on his symptoms and X-ray findings. Rather than immediately prescribing pain medications, the physician recommended a comprehensive approach following the ACR/AF guidelines.

The treatment plan began with patient education about OA and the importance of maintaining joint mobility. Robert learned that staying active was crucial for joint health, even though movement sometimes caused temporary discomfort. This understanding helped him overcome his fear of exercise.

Weight management became a priority since Robert had gained 30 pounds since retirement. Even modest weight loss could significantly reduce stress on his knees. He worked with a dietitian to develop a sustainable eating plan that created a moderate caloric deficit.

Physical therapy provided Robert with specific exercises to strengthen the muscles around his knees while improving flexibility. The program included low-impact activities like swimming and cycling that provided cardiovascular benefits without stressing his joints.

After six months of following this comprehensive approach, Robert's knee pain had decreased by 50%. He had lost 15 pounds and felt more confident in his ability to stay active. His case demonstrates how multimodal treatment can effectively manage OA symptoms while slowing disease progression.

## Exercise as Medicine for Osteoarthritis

Exercise represents one of the most effective treatments for OA, with benefits that often exceed those of medications. The key is choosing appropriate activities that strengthen muscles, maintain joint mobility, and provide cardiovascular benefits without causing additional joint damage.

Low-impact activities like swimming, cycling, and walking are ideal for people with OA. These activities provide exercise benefits while minimizing stress on affected joints. Water exercises are particularly beneficial because buoyancy reduces joint loading while providing resistance for muscle strengthening.

Strength training is crucial for OA management because strong muscles help stabilize joints and reduce stress on cartilage. The exercises should target muscles around affected joints, using resistance that challenges the muscles without causing excessive joint stress.

Flexibility and range-of-motion exercises help maintain joint mobility and reduce stiffness. These exercises should be performed daily, ideally after warming up with light activity. The goal is to maintain or improve joint flexibility rather than pushing through pain.

## Rheumatoid Arthritis and Integrative Approaches

Rheumatoid arthritis (RA) is an autoimmune condition that causes chronic inflammation in joints and other body systems. Unlike osteoarthritis, RA can affect people of any age and often causes systemic symptoms like fatigue and fever. Early diagnosis and treatment are crucial for preventing joint damage and disability.

The treatment of RA has been revolutionized by new medications that can effectively control inflammation and prevent joint damage. However, these medications work best when combined with lifestyle modifications and complementary therapies that address the whole person rather than just the disease.

**Case Example: Linda's Rheumatoid Arthritis Journey**

Linda, a 44-year-old marketing manager, developed joint pain and stiffness that initially appeared to be overuse injuries from her active lifestyle. However, when multiple joints became involved and she developed morning stiffness lasting several hours, her physician suspected RA.

Blood tests confirmed the diagnosis, showing elevated inflammatory markers and rheumatoid factor. Linda was initially overwhelmed by the diagnosis, fearing that she would become disabled and unable to maintain her active lifestyle.

Her rheumatologist explained that modern RA treatment could effectively control the disease and prevent joint damage. The treatment plan included disease-modifying antirheumatic drugs (DMARDs) to control inflammation, combined with lifestyle modifications to support overall health.

Linda began methotrexate, a DMARD that helps control the autoimmune process causing her joint inflammation. The medication required regular monitoring but provided significant improvement in her symptoms within a few months.

The integrative approach included stress management techniques because stress can worsen RA symptoms. Linda learned meditation and yoga, which helped her manage the anxiety about her diagnosis while providing gentle exercise that maintained joint mobility.

Dietary modifications focused on anti-inflammatory foods while avoiding potential trigger foods. Linda worked with a nutritionist to develop an eating plan rich in omega-3 fatty acids, antioxidants, and other nutrients that support immune function.

After one year of treatment, Linda's RA was in remission. She maintained her active lifestyle with some modifications and felt confident in her ability to manage her condition long-term. Her case illustrates how modern RA treatment can provide excellent outcomes when started early.

**The Role of Inflammation in RA**

RA involves chronic inflammation that affects not just joints but the entire body. This systemic inflammation can increase the risk of cardiovascular disease, osteoporosis, and other complications. Controlling inflammation is therefore crucial for both symptom management and long-term health.

Modern RA medications work by targeting specific components of the inflammatory process. Biological medications can block specific inflammatory chemicals, providing more targeted treatment than traditional anti-inflammatory drugs.

Lifestyle factors can significantly influence inflammation levels in RA. Stress, poor sleep, and inflammatory foods can worsen symptoms, while regular exercise, stress management, and anti-inflammatory nutrition can help control the disease.

**Joint-Friendly Exercise Prescriptions**

Exercise prescription for arthritis requires careful consideration of joint health, disease activity, and individual capabilities. The goal is to provide maximum benefit while minimizing the risk of joint damage or symptom flares.

**Low-Impact Cardiovascular Exercise**

Swimming and water aerobics provide excellent cardiovascular exercise while minimizing joint stress. The buoyancy of water reduces joint loading while providing resistance for muscle strengthening. Most people with arthritis can participate in water exercises regardless of disease severity.

Cycling, either stationary or outdoor, provides cardiovascular benefits while being gentle on joints. The smooth, circular motion is easier on joints than high-impact activities like running. Proper bike fit is important to avoid putting excessive stress on knees or hips.

Walking remains one of the best exercises for arthritis, but it should be done on appropriate surfaces with proper footwear. Treadmills can provide cushioning that reduces joint impact compared to concrete or asphalt surfaces.

### Strength Training Modifications

Strength training is crucial for people with arthritis, but it requires modifications to protect joints while building muscle. The focus should be on controlled movements through a full range of motion rather than maximum weight lifting.

Resistance bands provide variable resistance that can be adjusted to individual capabilities. They're particularly useful for people with hand or wrist arthritis because they don't require gripping heavy weights.

Isometric exercises involve muscle contraction without joint movement and can be particularly beneficial during arthritis flares when joint movement is painful. These exercises can maintain muscle strength even when traditional exercises are not tolerated.

### Case Example: Margaret's Exercise Success

Margaret, a 68-year-old with hip and knee osteoarthritis, had become increasingly sedentary due to pain and stiffness. She worried that exercise would worsen her arthritis and was hesitant to begin an exercise program.

Her physical therapist designed a progressive exercise program that started with gentle movements and gradually increased in intensity.

The program included pool exercises, which Margaret initially found easier than land-based activities.

The aquatic program included walking in shallow water, gentle leg swings, and arm movements that provided cardiovascular exercise while strengthening muscles. The warm water helped reduce stiffness and made movement more comfortable.

As Margaret's fitness improved, she added land-based exercises including strength training with resistance bands and balance activities. The program was adjusted based on her response, with modifications made during arthritis flares.

After six months, Margaret had improved significantly in both strength and endurance. Her arthritis pain had decreased, and she felt more confident in her ability to stay active. She continued the program long-term, viewing exercise as essential medicine for her arthritis.

## Dietary Interventions for Arthritis

Nutrition plays a significant role in arthritis management, with certain foods promoting inflammation while others help reduce it. The goal is to create an eating pattern that supports joint health while managing weight and overall health.

## Anti-Inflammatory Nutrition

The Mediterranean diet has strong research support for reducing inflammation and improving arthritis symptoms. This eating pattern emphasizes fruits, vegetables, whole grains, fish, and healthy fats while limiting processed foods and refined sugars.

Omega-3 fatty acids, found in fatty fish, walnuts, and flaxseeds, have potent anti-inflammatory effects. Regular consumption of these foods can help reduce joint inflammation and may allow for reduced medication use in some people.

Antioxidant-rich foods help combat oxidative stress that contributes to joint damage. Colorful fruits and vegetables provide diverse antioxidants that work together to reduce inflammation and support joint health.

**Foods to Limit or Avoid**

Processed foods, refined sugars, and trans fats can promote inflammation and worsen arthritis symptoms. These foods should be minimized in favor of whole, unprocessed options that provide better nutrition and less inflammatory potential.

Some people with arthritis may benefit from avoiding nightshade vegetables (tomatoes, peppers, eggplant, potatoes), though scientific evidence for this is limited. Individual food sensitivities can be identified through elimination diets if suspected.

Excessive alcohol consumption can interfere with arthritis medications and may worsen inflammation. Moderate consumption may be acceptable for some people, but this should be discussed with healthcare providers.

**Case Example: Thomas's Dietary Transformation**

Thomas, a 58-year-old with rheumatoid arthritis, noticed that his symptoms seemed to fluctuate with his diet. He decided to work with a registered dietitian to identify foods that might be triggering his symptoms.

The dietitian helped Thomas transition to a Mediterranean-style eating pattern while keeping a food and symptom diary. This approach allowed him to identify patterns between his diet and arthritis symptoms.

Thomas discovered that processed foods and excess sugar consistently worsened his joint pain and stiffness. He eliminated these foods and focused on whole, anti-inflammatory options including fatty fish, leafy greens, and colorful vegetables.

The dietary changes complemented his medical treatment and helped him achieve better symptom control. His inflammatory markers improved, and he felt more energetic and less stiff. Thomas continued the eating plan long-term, viewing it as an essential part of his arthritis management.

## Protecting Your Joints for Long-Term Health

Joint protection strategies can slow arthritis progression and improve quality of life. These approaches focus on reducing joint stress while maintaining function and independence.

## Ergonomic Modifications

Simple modifications to daily activities can significantly reduce joint stress. Using larger, stronger joints for tasks reduces stress on smaller, more vulnerable joints. For example, carrying bags with shoulder straps rather than handles reduces stress on finger joints.

Adaptive equipment can help people with arthritis maintain independence while protecting joints. Jar openers, ergonomic tools, and built-up handles on utensils can make daily tasks easier and less stressful on joints.

Proper body mechanics during daily activities can prevent excessive joint stress. This includes maintaining good posture, using proper lifting techniques, and avoiding prolonged positions that stress joints.

## Weight Management

Excess weight puts additional stress on weight-bearing joints, particularly knees and hips. Even modest weight loss can provide significant benefits for arthritis symptoms and slow disease progression.

The relationship between weight and arthritis is particularly strong for knee osteoarthritis. Each pound of weight loss reduces knee stress by approximately four pounds during walking, making weight management a powerful tool for symptom relief.

Sustainable weight loss requires a comprehensive approach that includes dietary changes, increased physical activity, and behavioral modifications. The goal should be gradual, sustained weight loss rather than rapid changes that are difficult to maintain.

## Activity Modification

Balancing activity with rest is crucial for arthritis management. Overdoing activities can cause symptom flares, while too little activity can lead to stiffness and weakness. The goal is finding the right balance for each individual.

Pacing activities throughout the day can help prevent overuse and fatigue. This might involve alternating between different types of activities or taking breaks before fatigue sets in.

Modifying high-impact activities to lower-impact alternatives can allow people with arthritis to stay active while protecting joints. For example, switching from running to swimming or cycling can provide similar cardiovascular benefits with less joint stress.

## Building Your Arthritis Management Team

Effective arthritis management often requires a team approach involving multiple healthcare providers. Each team member brings specialized knowledge and skills that contribute to optimal outcomes.

## Primary Care Coordination

Primary care physicians often serve as the coordinator for arthritis care, managing overall health while referring to specialists when needed. They can monitor for complications, adjust medications, and ensure that all aspects of health are addressed.

## Specialist Involvement

Rheumatologists specialize in arthritis and autoimmune conditions and are essential for managing complex cases. They have expertise in the latest medications and treatment approaches and can provide specialized care that primary care physicians may not offer.

Physical therapists provide exercise prescription and manual therapy techniques that can improve joint function and reduce pain. They can design individualized programs that address specific limitations and goals.

Occupational therapists focus on daily activities and can recommend adaptive equipment and techniques that reduce joint stress while maintaining independence. They're particularly helpful for people with hand and wrist arthritis.

## The Road Ahead

Arthritis management continues to evolve with new medications, treatment approaches, and understanding of disease mechanisms. The key to successful management lies in early intervention, comprehensive care, and active patient participation in treatment decisions.

The next chapter will explore fibromyalgia and widespread pain conditions, which often coexist with arthritis and require specialized approaches for optimal management.

## Joint Health Foundations

Arthritis management has progressed from a focus on symptom control to comprehensive care that addresses function, quality of life, and disease progression. The evidence supports multimodal approaches that combine appropriate medications with lifestyle modifications and complementary therapies.

Success in arthritis management requires patience, persistence, and active participation in treatment decisions. The goal is not just pain relief but maintaining function and quality of life throughout the course of the disease.

## Core Arthritis Management Principles:

- Evidence-based guidelines support multimodal approaches combining drug and non-drug treatments

- Exercise is essential medicine for arthritis, with benefits that often exceed those of medications

- Anti-inflammatory nutrition can significantly impact arthritis symptoms and disease progression

- Joint protection strategies can slow arthritis progression while maintaining function

- Weight management provides powerful benefits for arthritis symptoms and long-term outcomes

- Team-based care optimizes outcomes by addressing all aspects of arthritis management

# Chapter 12: Fibromyalgia and Widespread Pain

Fibromyalgia challenges everything we traditionally understand about pain. This condition affects 2-4% of the population, primarily women, and creates widespread pain without visible injury or inflammation. For decades, fibromyalgia was dismissed as psychological or imaginary, leaving millions of people suffering without adequate care. Today, we understand fibromyalgia as a real neurological condition involving central sensitization - changes in how the nervous system processes pain signals.

The American Academy of Family Physicians has published comprehensive guidelines for fibromyalgia management that acknowledge the condition's complexity and the need for multimodal treatment approaches (79, 80). These guidelines represent a significant shift from symptom-focused care to comprehensive management that addresses the multiple dimensions of fibromyalgia.

**Understanding Central Sensitization**

Central sensitization is the key to understanding fibromyalgia and other widespread pain conditions. This process involves changes in the central nervous system that make it hypersensitive to pain signals. The result is a condition where normal sensations become painful and pain signals are amplified throughout the body.

Think of central sensitization as a car alarm system that's become too sensitive. Instead of only responding to actual threats like break-ins, it now goes off when someone walks by, when the wind blows, or even when nothing is happening at all. Similarly, in fibromyalgia, the pain system responds to normal sensations as if they were threats, creating pain where none should exist.

This understanding helps explain why fibromyalgia pain doesn't follow typical patterns. The pain can move around the body, vary in intensity without clear triggers, and affect multiple body systems simultaneously. It's not that the pain is imaginary - it's that the pain processing system has become hypersensitive.

**Case Example: Sarah's Fibromyalgia Journey**

Sarah, a 42-year-old office manager, developed widespread pain that began gradually after a stressful period at work. Initially, she attributed the pain to poor posture and long hours at her desk. However, the pain spread throughout her body and was accompanied by fatigue, sleep problems, and cognitive difficulties.

Multiple medical evaluations found no obvious cause for Sarah's symptoms. Blood tests were normal, imaging studies showed no abnormalities, and various specialists couldn't identify a specific condition. Sarah began to worry that she was "going crazy" or that her symptoms were psychological.

Finally, a rheumatologist diagnosed fibromyalgia based on Sarah's symptom pattern and physical examination. The diagnosis was both a relief and a challenge - relief because she finally had an explanation for her symptoms, but challenging because she learned that fibromyalgia is a chronic condition requiring ongoing management.

The physician explained central sensitization and how it created Sarah's symptoms. This understanding helped her realize that her pain was real and had a biological basis. She learned that fibromyalgia isn't progressive or life-threatening, but it does require active management.

Sarah's treatment plan addressed multiple aspects of fibromyalgia including pain management, sleep improvement, and stress reduction. She began low-dose antidepressant medication that helped normalize her sleep and reduce pain sensitivity.

The treatment also included a gradual exercise program designed specifically for fibromyalgia. Sarah started with gentle stretching and walking, gradually building her tolerance for activity. The key was starting slowly and progressing gradually to avoid triggering symptom flares.

After six months of treatment, Sarah's pain had decreased by 40% and her sleep quality had improved significantly. She felt more in control of her condition and had developed skills for managing flares when they occurred. Her case illustrates how understanding fibromyalgia can lead to effective management.

## The Three Pillars of Fibromyalgia Treatment

The American Academy of Family Physicians identifies three main pillars of fibromyalgia treatment: exercise, cognitive behavioral therapy, and appropriate medication (81). This tripartite approach addresses the multiple aspects of fibromyalgia and provides the best outcomes for most people.

## Exercise as Foundation

Exercise is perhaps the most important treatment for fibromyalgia, though it must be approached carefully. People with fibromyalgia often have exercise intolerance and may experience increased pain after activity. However, gradual, appropriate exercise can significantly improve symptoms and quality of life.

The key to exercise success in fibromyalgia is starting at a very low intensity and progressing slowly. Many people with fibromyalgia have been sedentary due to pain and fatigue, making their tolerance for exercise very low. The goal is to gradually rebuild fitness without triggering major symptom flares.

Aerobic exercise appears to be particularly beneficial for fibromyalgia. Low-impact activities like walking, swimming, and cycling can improve cardiovascular fitness while reducing pain sensitivity. The exercise should be performed at moderate intensity - enough to provide benefit without causing exhaustion.

Strength training can also be beneficial for fibromyalgia, though it should be introduced gradually after establishing aerobic fitness. Building muscle strength can improve daily function and may help reduce pain sensitivity over time.

## Cognitive Behavioral Therapy

CBT for fibromyalgia focuses on changing thought patterns and behaviors that contribute to pain and disability. People with fibromyalgia often develop catastrophic thinking patterns about their symptoms, which can increase pain intensity and emotional distress.

The therapy helps people identify and challenge unhelpful thoughts about pain and develop more balanced perspectives. For example, instead of thinking "this pain will never end," people learn to think "this is a temporary flare that will improve."

CBT also addresses behavioral factors that can worsen fibromyalgia symptoms. This includes activity pacing, stress management, and sleep hygiene. People learn to balance activity with rest and develop strategies for managing stress.

## Medication Management

Medication plays a supporting role in fibromyalgia treatment, with several FDA-approved options available. These medications work by modulating pain processing in the nervous system rather than treating inflammation or tissue damage.

Pregabalin was the first medication specifically approved for fibromyalgia. It works by reducing the release of neurotransmitters that contribute to pain signaling. The medication can provide significant pain relief for some people, though side effects like dizziness and weight gain can be problematic.

Duloxetine and milnacipran are antidepressants that have been approved for fibromyalgia. These medications work by increasing levels of serotonin and norepinephrine, neurotransmitters that help regulate pain and mood. They can provide pain relief even in people who aren't depressed.

## Pacing and Energy Management

The "spoon theory" provides a useful framework for understanding and managing energy in fibromyalgia. Developed by Christine Miserandino, who has lupus, the theory uses spoons as a metaphor for energy units. Each person starts the day with a limited number of spoons, and every activity costs spoons.

People with fibromyalgia often have fewer spoons than healthy individuals, and they may use spoons more quickly for the same activities. Understanding this helps explain why someone with fibromyalgia might feel exhausted after activities that seem simple to others.

## Case Example: Jennifer's Pacing Success

Jennifer, a 38-year-old teacher with fibromyalgia, struggled with the boom-bust cycle common in chronic pain conditions. On good days, she would try to catch up on everything she couldn't do on bad days, often triggering severe symptom flares.

Jennifer learned about pacing and energy management through a fibromyalgia support group. She began tracking her energy levels and activities to identify patterns. She discovered that pushing herself on good days consistently led to several days of increased symptoms.

The pacing strategy involved dividing large tasks into smaller components and spreading them across multiple days. Instead of cleaning the entire house in one day, Jennifer would clean one room per day, allowing her to maintain her home without exhausting herself.

Jennifer also learned to alternate between high-energy and low-energy activities throughout the day. After a demanding work meeting, she would schedule a less demanding activity to allow her energy to recover. This approach helped prevent the energy crashes that had previously triggered symptom flares.

The pacing strategy required Jennifer to adjust her expectations and accept that she might not accomplish as much as she previously did. However, she found that consistent, moderate activity levels actually allowed her to accomplish more over time than the previous boom-bust pattern.

### Activity Modification Strategies

Successful pacing involves more than just limiting activity - it requires strategic planning and modification of activities to conserve energy while maintaining function. This might involve using assistive devices, changing work methods, or rescheduling activities.

Prioritization becomes crucial when energy is limited. People with fibromyalgia must learn to identify which activities are most important and focus their energy on those priorities. This might mean saying no to some activities to preserve energy for others.

Planning ahead can help distribute energy more effectively. This might involve preparing meals in advance, organizing workspace to reduce movement, or scheduling demanding activities during times when energy is typically higher.

### Sleep Restoration and Fibromyalgia

Sleep problems are nearly universal in fibromyalgia, and addressing these issues is crucial for symptom management. People with fibromyalgia often experience non-restorative sleep - they may sleep for adequate hours but wake up feeling unrefreshed and tired.

The relationship between sleep and fibromyalgia is bidirectional. Poor sleep can worsen pain and fatigue, while pain and other symptoms can disrupt sleep quality. Breaking this cycle requires addressing both sleep hygiene and pain management.

### Sleep Architecture in Fibromyalgia

Research has shown that people with fibromyalgia have abnormal sleep architecture, with frequent interruptions of deep sleep stages. This disruption prevents the restorative processes that normally occur during sleep, contributing to pain and fatigue.

The sleep problems in fibromyalgia are not just about quantity but quality. People may spend adequate time in bed but not achieve the deep, restorative sleep necessary for healing and recovery. This explains why people with fibromyalgia often wake up feeling tired despite sleeping for many hours.

## Case Example: Michael's Sleep Transformation

Michael, a 45-year-old with fibromyalgia, struggled with severe sleep problems that worsened his other symptoms. He would often lie awake for hours before falling asleep, then wake up frequently during the night. He felt exhausted every morning regardless of how many hours he spent in bed.

Michael's physician prescribed a low-dose tricyclic antidepressant specifically for its sleep-promoting effects. The medication helped him fall asleep more easily and stay asleep longer. However, medication alone wasn't sufficient to address all his sleep problems.

The sleep improvement plan also included strict sleep hygiene measures. Michael established a consistent bedtime routine, avoided screens before bed, and kept his bedroom cool and dark. He also eliminated caffeine after 2 PM and avoided large meals close to bedtime.

Michael learned relaxation techniques specifically for bedtime, including progressive muscle relaxation and guided imagery. These techniques helped calm his nervous system and prepare his body for sleep. He practiced these techniques consistently, even when he didn't feel like they were helping immediately.

After three months of comprehensive sleep treatment, Michael's sleep quality had improved dramatically. He was falling asleep more quickly, staying asleep longer, and waking up more refreshed. The improved sleep had a positive impact on his pain levels and overall quality of life.

## Building Your Fibromyalgia Support Team

Fibromyalgia management requires a multidisciplinary approach involving various healthcare providers and support systems. Each team member brings specialized knowledge and skills that contribute to optimal outcomes.

## Medical Team Coordination

Primary care physicians often serve as the coordinator for fibromyalgia care, managing overall health while referring to specialists when needed. They can monitor for complications, adjust medications, and ensure that all aspects of health are addressed.

Rheumatologists have specialized knowledge of fibromyalgia and can provide expert diagnosis and treatment. They're particularly helpful for complex cases or when the diagnosis is uncertain.

Pain management specialists can provide additional treatment options for people with severe or treatment-resistant fibromyalgia. They may offer specialized procedures or medication combinations that aren't available through primary care.

## Psychological Support

Mental health professionals play a crucial role in fibromyalgia management. Chronic pain conditions can contribute to depression and anxiety, which can worsen fibromyalgia symptoms. Addressing these psychological factors is essential for optimal outcomes.

Cognitive behavioral therapy specifically designed for chronic pain can provide valuable skills for managing fibromyalgia. These therapists understand the unique challenges of chronic pain and can provide targeted interventions.

## Alternative and Complementary Practitioners

Many people with fibromyalgia benefit from complementary approaches like acupuncture, massage therapy, and chiropractic care. These treatments can provide additional pain relief and may help address specific symptoms.

Physical therapists can design exercise programs specifically for fibromyalgia and provide education about activity pacing. They understand the unique challenges of exercising with fibromyalgia and can provide modifications to prevent symptom flares.

## Support Groups and Peer Support

Connecting with others who have fibromyalgia can provide emotional support and practical advice. Support groups, both in-person and online, can help people feel less isolated and learn from others' experiences.

Peer support can be particularly valuable for learning practical management strategies. People with fibromyalgia often develop creative solutions for daily challenges, and sharing these strategies can benefit others.

## Living Well with Fibromyalgia

Fibromyalgia is a chronic condition that requires ongoing management, but many people are able to live full, productive lives with appropriate treatment. The key is accepting the condition while actively working to manage symptoms and maintain function.

Success with fibromyalgia often involves adjusting expectations and finding new ways to accomplish goals. This might mean working part-time instead of full-time, or finding different ways to participate in enjoyable activities.

The next chapter will explore headaches and migraines, conditions that often coexist with fibromyalgia and require specialized approaches for optimal management.

## Widespread Pain Wisdom

Fibromyalgia represents a paradigm shift in our understanding of pain - from a simple signal of tissue damage to a complex neurological condition involving central sensitization. This understanding has led to more effective treatments that address the underlying mechanisms rather than just symptoms.

The three-pillar approach of exercise, CBT, and appropriate medication provides a framework for comprehensive fibromyalgia management. Success requires patience, persistence, and a willingness to try different approaches to find what works best for each individual.

**Fibromyalgia Management Essentials:**

- Central sensitization explains why fibromyalgia pain doesn't follow typical patterns

- The three pillars of treatment - exercise, CBT, and medication - address multiple aspects of the condition

- Pacing and energy management using the spoon theory prevents boom-bust cycles

- Sleep restoration is crucial for fibromyalgia management and requires comprehensive approaches

- Multidisciplinary care teams provide the best outcomes for complex fibromyalgia cases

- Living well with fibromyalgia requires accepting the condition while actively managing symptoms

# Chapter 13: Headaches and Migraines

Headaches strike nearly everyone at some point, but for millions of Americans, they represent a chronic, debilitating condition that significantly impacts quality of life. Migraines alone affect 39 million Americans, with women three times more likely to be affected than men. Yet despite their prevalence, headaches and migraines are often undertreated, leaving people suffering unnecessarily when effective treatments are available.

The landscape of headache treatment has been revolutionized by advances in understanding migraine mechanisms and the development of targeted therapies. New medications, innovative devices, and evidence-based lifestyle approaches now offer hope for people who previously had few options for relief.

## Understanding Your Headache Patterns

Effective headache management begins with understanding your specific headache type and triggers. Not all headaches are the same, and different types require different treatment approaches. The key is becoming a detective in your own health, identifying patterns that can guide treatment decisions.

Primary headaches, including migraines, tension headaches, and cluster headaches, occur without underlying disease. Secondary headaches result from other conditions like infections, medication overuse, or structural problems. Distinguishing between these types is crucial for appropriate treatment.

## Migraine Characteristics

Migraines are complex neurological events that involve more than just head pain. They typically cause throbbing, pulsating pain on one side of the head, though they can affect both sides. The pain is often accompanied by nausea, vomiting, and sensitivity to light and sound.

Many people experience warning signs before migraine attacks, including mood changes, food cravings, or neck stiffness. Some people experience aura - visual disturbances like flashing lights or zigzag patterns - before the headache phase begins.

Migraines can last anywhere from four hours to several days if untreated. The frequency varies widely, with some people experiencing occasional attacks while others have chronic daily migraines. Understanding your personal migraine pattern is essential for effective treatment.

## Case Example: Lisa's Migraine Detective Work

Lisa, a 34-year-old attorney, suffered from severe migraines that were disrupting her career and personal life. The headaches seemed to strike randomly, lasting 2-3 days and leaving her unable to work or care for her family.

Lisa's neurologist recommended keeping a detailed headache diary to identify patterns and triggers. She tracked everything: what she ate, how she slept, her stress levels, weather changes, and her menstrual cycle. Initially, the task felt overwhelming, but patterns began to emerge.

Lisa discovered that her migraines were strongly linked to her menstrual cycle, typically occurring 2-3 days before her period. She also identified several food triggers, including aged cheeses and red wine. Stress at work and inadequate sleep also seemed to precipitate attacks.

Weather changes, particularly drops in barometric pressure, consistently triggered Lisa's migraines. While she couldn't control the weather, understanding this trigger helped her prepare for potential attacks by ensuring she had medication available and could adjust her schedule if needed.

Armed with this information, Lisa worked with her neurologist to develop a comprehensive prevention plan. She started hormonal therapy to stabilize her menstrual cycle, eliminated known food triggers, and implemented stress management techniques.

The migraine diary also revealed that Lisa's attacks followed a predictable pattern, allowing her to use acute medications more effectively. By taking medication at the first sign of a migraine, she could often prevent it from becoming severe.

After six months of pattern recognition and targeted treatment, Lisa's migraine frequency had decreased by 70%. The attacks that did occur were less severe and more manageable. Her case demonstrates how understanding personal headache patterns can transform treatment outcomes.

## Prevention Protocols and CGRP Therapies

Migraine prevention has been revolutionized by the development of medications targeting calcitonin gene-related peptide (CGRP), a protein involved in migraine pathways. These medications represent the first treatments specifically developed for migraine prevention, offering new hope for people with frequent attacks.

The American Headache Society has published updated guidance on migraine prevention therapy, incorporating these new CGRP medications into treatment algorithms (82). The guidelines emphasize that prevention should be considered for people with frequent migraines or those that significantly impact quality of life.

## CGRP Inhibitors

CGRP inhibitors work by blocking the action of CGRP, a protein that plays a key role in migraine development. These medications are administered as monthly or quarterly injections and can significantly reduce migraine frequency and severity.

The medications are generally well-tolerated, with fewer side effects than traditional migraine preventive medications. Common side effects include injection site reactions and constipation, but serious adverse effects are rare.

Clinical trials have shown that CGRP inhibitors can reduce migraine frequency by 50% or more in many people. The medications are particularly beneficial for people who haven't responded to other preventive treatments or who can't tolerate traditional medications.

## Traditional Preventive Medications

Before CGRP inhibitors, migraine prevention relied on medications originally developed for other conditions. These include blood pressure medications, antidepressants, and anti-seizure drugs. While effective for many people, these medications often cause side effects that limit their use.

Propranolol, a beta-blocker, remains one of the most effective migraine preventive medications. It can reduce migraine frequency by 50% or more in many people, though it may cause fatigue and can affect heart rate and blood pressure.

Topiramate, an anti-seizure medication, is another effective preventive option. However, it can cause cognitive side effects, kidney stones, and weight loss, making it unsuitable for some people.

## Case Example: Robert's Prevention Success

Robert, a 48-year-old teacher, experienced migraines 15-20 days per month, making it difficult to maintain his teaching schedule. Traditional acute treatments provided limited relief, and he was becoming dependent on pain medications.

His neurologist recommended starting preventive treatment with a CGRP inhibitor. Robert was initially hesitant about monthly injections but agreed to try the treatment given his frequent migraines.

The CGRP inhibitor was administered as a monthly injection that Robert learned to give himself. The treatment was surprisingly easy, and he experienced no significant side effects. The improvement in his migraines was gradual but substantial.

After three months of treatment, Robert's migraine frequency had decreased from 15-20 days per month to 5-8 days per month. The migraines that did occur were less severe and more responsive to acute treatments.

Robert also implemented lifestyle modifications including regular sleep schedules, stress management, and trigger avoidance. The combination of medication and lifestyle changes allowed him to return to full-time teaching without missing work due to migraines.

His case illustrates how modern preventive treatments can transform the lives of people with frequent migraines. The CGRP inhibitor provided benefits that weren't achievable with traditional preventive medications.

## Acute Treatment Without Opioids

Effective acute migraine treatment focuses on stopping attacks quickly while avoiding medication overuse. The goal is to treat migraines early and effectively, preventing them from becoming severe and disabling.

Research published in Medscape and PubMed has documented the effectiveness of various non-opioid acute treatments for migraines (83, 84). These treatments work through different mechanisms and can be combined for optimal effect.

## Triptans

Triptans are medications specifically designed to treat migraines and represent the gold standard for acute treatment. They work by constricting blood vessels and blocking pain pathways in the brain. Seven different triptans are available, allowing for individualized treatment.

Sumatriptan was the first triptan developed and remains widely used. It's available in multiple formulations including tablets, injections, and nasal spray. The injection provides the fastest relief but may cause more side effects.

Newer triptans like rizatriptan and eletriptan may be more effective or better tolerated than sumatriptan for some people. The key is finding the right triptan and formulation for each individual's needs.

## CGRP Receptor Antagonists

Oral CGRP receptor antagonists provide a new option for acute migraine treatment. These medications work by blocking CGRP receptors during migraine attacks, providing relief without the vascular effects of triptans.

Ubrogepant and rimegepant are two CGRP receptor antagonists approved for acute migraine treatment. They may be particularly useful for people who can't use triptans due to cardiovascular concerns.

## Combination Therapies

Many people benefit from combining different acute treatments. For example, a triptan might be combined with an anti-nausea medication and a non-steroidal anti-inflammatory drug (NSAID) for comprehensive symptom relief.

The combination of sumatriptan and naproxen is available as a single tablet and has been shown to be more effective than either medication alone. This combination addresses both pain and inflammation associated with migraines.

## Case Example: Patricia's Acute Treatment Evolution

Patricia, a 29-year-old graphic designer, struggled with severe migraines that would leave her bedridden for days. Over-the-counter medications provided minimal relief, and she was concerned about using prescription pain medications.

Her physician prescribed sumatriptan for acute treatment. Patricia was initially wary of prescription medications but agreed to try the treatment given her severe symptoms. The first time she used sumatriptan, she was amazed by its effectiveness.

The sumatriptan provided significant relief within 30 minutes of taking it. However, Patricia discovered that it worked best when taken at the first sign of a migraine rather than waiting for the pain to become severe.

Patricia also learned to combine the sumatriptan with an anti-nausea medication and ibuprofen for more comprehensive relief. This combination approach addressed all aspects of her migraines and provided more complete symptom control.

Over time, Patricia developed a personalized acute treatment plan that included recognizing early warning signs, taking medication promptly, and creating a supportive environment for recovery. This approach reduced her migraine disability significantly.

## Lifestyle Medicine for Headaches

Lifestyle factors play a crucial role in headache management, with diet, sleep, and stress being particularly important. These factors can serve as both triggers and treatments, making lifestyle modification an essential component of headache management.

## Sleep and Headaches

Sleep disturbances are both triggers and consequences of headaches. Poor sleep quality can precipitate headaches, while headaches can disrupt sleep, creating a vicious cycle. Addressing sleep issues is therefore crucial for headache management.

Maintaining consistent sleep schedules helps regulate circadian rhythms and may reduce headache frequency. This means going to bed and waking up at the same time every day, even on weekends.

Sleep hygiene measures include creating a dark, quiet, cool sleeping environment and avoiding screens before bedtime. These measures can improve sleep quality and may reduce headache frequency.

## Stress Management

Stress is one of the most common headache triggers, and chronic stress can increase headache frequency and severity. Effective stress management is therefore essential for headache prevention.

Relaxation techniques like progressive muscle relaxation, deep breathing, and meditation can help reduce stress and may prevent headaches. These techniques work best when practiced regularly rather than just during stressful periods.

Time management and lifestyle modifications can help reduce chronic stress. This might involve setting boundaries, delegating responsibilities, or making changes to reduce daily stressors.

## Dietary Factors

Certain foods can trigger headaches in susceptible individuals. Common triggers include aged cheeses, processed meats, alcohol, and foods containing MSG. Identifying and avoiding personal triggers can reduce headache frequency.

Skipping meals can also trigger headaches, making regular eating patterns important for headache prevention. Maintaining stable blood sugar levels through regular meals and snacks can help prevent headaches.

Adequate hydration is essential for headache prevention. Dehydration is a common headache trigger, and maintaining proper fluid intake can help prevent attacks.

## Neuromodulation Options

Advanced technological approaches to headache treatment include various forms of neuromodulation - treatments that modify nerve activity to reduce pain. These approaches offer alternatives for people who don't respond to traditional treatments.

## Non-Invasive Neuromodulation

Transcutaneous electrical nerve stimulation (TENS) devices designed specifically for headaches can provide relief for some people. These devices deliver electrical stimulation to nerve pathways involved in headache pain.

Transcranial magnetic stimulation (TMS) uses magnetic fields to stimulate specific brain regions involved in migraine. This treatment is available for acute migraine treatment and may be particularly useful for people who experience aura.

## Invasive Neuromodulation

Occipital nerve stimulation involves implanting electrodes near nerves at the back of the head. This treatment may be considered for people with severe, treatment-resistant headaches.

Sphenopalatine ganglion stimulation targets a nerve cluster involved in headache pain. This treatment requires surgical implantation but may provide significant relief for people with cluster headaches or severe migraines.

## Building Your Headache Management Plan

Effective headache management requires a personalized approach that addresses your specific headache type, triggers, and treatment response. The plan should include both acute and preventive strategies tailored to your individual needs.

## Tracking and Monitoring

Keeping a headache diary helps identify patterns and triggers while monitoring treatment effectiveness. The diary should include headache frequency, severity, triggers, treatments used, and response to treatment.

Many smartphone apps are available for headache tracking, making it easier to maintain consistent records. These apps often include features like weather tracking and medication reminders.

## Treatment Escalation

Having a clear plan for different levels of headache severity helps ensure appropriate treatment. This might include different medications for mild versus severe headaches, or specific steps to take when usual treatments aren't effective.

## Medication Management

Avoiding medication overuse is crucial for headache management. Overuse of acute medications can lead to rebound headaches and increased headache frequency. Clear guidelines for medication use help prevent this problem.

## The Path Forward

Headache management has been transformed by advances in understanding migraine mechanisms and the development of targeted therapies. The availability of CGRP-based treatments offers new hope for people with frequent or severe headaches.

The next chapter will explore neuropathic pain conditions, which require different approaches than the headache and migraine treatments discussed here.

## Headache Treatment Insights

Modern headache management combines targeted medications with lifestyle modifications and advanced technologies to provide comprehensive relief. The key is understanding your personal headache patterns and developing an individualized treatment plan.

Success in headache management often requires patience and persistence. Finding the right combination of treatments may take time, but the potential for significant improvement is greater than ever before.

## Headache Management Fundamentals:

- Understanding headache patterns and triggers is essential for effective treatment

- CGRP-based therapies have revolutionized both acute and preventive migraine treatment

- Non-opioid acute treatments can effectively stop migraines when used appropriately

- Lifestyle modifications addressing sleep, stress, and diet are crucial for headache prevention

- Neuromodulation options provide alternatives for treatment-resistant cases

- Personalized treatment plans combining multiple approaches optimize headache management outcomes

# Chapter 14: Neuropathic Pain and CRPS

Neuropathic pain represents one of the most challenging forms of chronic pain, affecting millions of Americans with conditions ranging from diabetic neuropathy to complex regional pain syndrome (CRPS). Unlike nociceptive pain that results from tissue damage, neuropathic pain arises from dysfunction in the nervous system itself. This fundamental difference means that traditional pain treatments often fail, leaving people struggling with burning, shooting, or electric shock-like sensations that can be debilitating.

Understanding neuropathic pain requires grasping that the nervous system, which normally processes and transmits pain signals, has become part of the problem. Damaged or dysfunctional nerves generate abnormal signals that the brain interprets as pain, even when no tissue damage exists. This mechanism explains why neuropathic pain often feels so different from other types of pain and why it requires specialized treatment approaches.

**Understanding Nerve Pain Mechanisms**

Neuropathic pain develops through several mechanisms that distinguish it from other forms of pain. Peripheral sensitization occurs when damaged nerves become hyperexcitable, generating spontaneous pain signals. Central sensitization involves changes in the spinal cord and brain that amplify these abnormal signals, making them feel more intense.

The quality of neuropathic pain often provides clues about its underlying mechanisms. Burning pain typically suggests involvement of small nerve fibers, while shooting or electric shock-like pain often indicates damage to larger nerve fibers. Allodynia - pain from normally non-painful stimuli like light touch - suggests central sensitization.

**Types of Neuropathic Pain**

Diabetic neuropathy is the most common form of neuropathic pain, affecting up to 50% of people with diabetes. The condition typically begins in the feet and hands, causing burning, tingling, or shooting pain. The pain is often worse at night and can significantly impact sleep quality.

Postherpetic neuralgia develops after shingles and can persist for months or years after the rash heals. The pain is typically burning or stabbing and may be accompanied by severe allodynia. This condition is more common in older adults and can be particularly debilitating.

Trigeminal neuralgia causes severe, electric shock-like pain in the face. The pain is typically triggered by light touch and can be so severe that people avoid eating, speaking, or touching their face. This condition is often described as one of the most painful conditions known to medicine.

**Case Example: David's Diabetic Neuropathy Journey**

David, a 58-year-old construction worker, developed type 2 diabetes that was initially well-controlled with medication and lifestyle changes. However, after several years, he began experiencing burning pain in his feet that gradually worsened and spread up his legs.

Initially, David attributed the pain to his physically demanding job and tried over-the-counter pain medications. However, the pain persisted and worsened, particularly at night. The burning sensation was so intense that even bed sheets touching his feet caused severe pain.

David's physician diagnosed diabetic neuropathy and explained that the high blood sugar levels over time had damaged the nerves in his feet. The pain wasn't coming from injured tissue but from the damaged nerves themselves, which explained why traditional pain medications weren't effective.

The treatment plan focused on better blood sugar control to prevent further nerve damage, combined with medications specifically designed for neuropathic pain. David was started on gabapentin, which helped reduce the burning pain but caused some dizziness and fatigue.

David also learned about the importance of foot care and inspection, as diabetic neuropathy can reduce sensation and increase the risk of injuries. He began checking his feet daily and wearing proper footwear to prevent complications.

After several months of treatment, David's pain had decreased by about 60%. While not completely pain-free, he was able to sleep better and maintain his work activities. His case illustrates how neuropathic pain requires specialized approaches different from other types of pain.

### First-Line Treatments for Neuropathic Pain

The treatment of neuropathic pain has evolved significantly with the development of medications that target the specific mechanisms involved in nerve pain. The NCBI has published extensive research on various treatment options for neuropathic pain conditions (85, 86, 87, 88, 89).

### Gabapentinoids

Gabapentin and pregabalin are the most commonly prescribed medications for neuropathic pain. These drugs work by binding to calcium channels in nerve cells, reducing the release of neurotransmitters that contribute to pain signals.

Gabapentin is typically started at a low dose and gradually increased to minimize side effects. Common side effects include dizziness, drowsiness, and swelling. The medication is generally well-tolerated, but some people experience cognitive side effects that can be problematic.

Pregabalin works through a similar mechanism but may be more effective for some people. It's also associated with fewer drug interactions than gabapentin. However, pregabalin is more expensive and may cause weight gain in some people.

### Antidepressants

Certain antidepressants are effective for neuropathic pain, even in people who aren't depressed. These medications work by increasing levels of neurotransmitters like serotonin and norepinephrine that help regulate pain signals.

Tricyclic antidepressants like amitriptyline and nortriptyline are particularly effective for neuropathic pain. However, they can cause side effects like dry mouth, constipation, and sedation. These medications are typically started at low doses and taken at bedtime.

Newer antidepressants like duloxetine and venlafaxine may be better tolerated than tricyclics while providing similar pain relief. These medications are particularly useful for people who also have depression or anxiety.

**Topical Treatments**

Topical medications can provide localized pain relief with fewer systemic side effects. Lidocaine patches are FDA-approved for postherpetic neuralgia and can provide significant relief for localized neuropathic pain.

Capsaicin cream, derived from chili peppers, can help reduce neuropathic pain by depleting substance P, a neurotransmitter involved in pain transmission. The cream may cause initial burning but can provide long-lasting relief with regular use.

**Case Example: Maria's Postherpetic Neuralgia Treatment**

Maria, a 72-year-old retiree, developed shingles on her left side that healed after several weeks. However, she continued to experience severe burning pain in the area where the rash had been. The pain was so intense that she couldn't tolerate clothing touching the affected skin.

Her physician diagnosed postherpetic neuralgia and explained that the shingles virus had damaged the nerves, causing ongoing pain even after the infection cleared. The pain was neuropathic rather than from tissue damage, requiring specialized treatment.

Maria was started on gabapentin, which provided some relief but caused significant drowsiness. Her physician adjusted the dosing schedule and added a lidocaine patch for localized relief. The combination provided better pain control with fewer side effects.

Maria also learned about the importance of protecting the affected skin from irritation. She wore loose-fitting clothing and used topical treatments to reduce nerve sensitivity. These strategies helped make her daily activities more tolerable.

After several months of treatment, Maria's pain had decreased significantly. While not completely pain-free, she was able to resume most of her normal activities. Her case demonstrates how combination treatments can effectively manage neuropathic pain.

## Desensitization Techniques

Desensitization involves gradually exposing hypersensitive nerves to stimuli to reduce their reactivity. This approach is particularly useful for conditions involving allodynia, where normally non-painful stimuli cause pain.

## Graded Exposure Therapy

Graded exposure begins with stimuli that are tolerable and gradually progresses to more challenging ones. For someone with allodynia, this might begin with gentle touch using soft materials and progress to firmer pressure over time.

The process requires patience and consistency. The goal is to retrain the nervous system to respond normally to sensory input rather than interpreting everything as painful. This retraining process can take weeks or months to achieve significant benefits.

## Sensory Retraining

Sensory retraining involves specific exercises designed to normalize sensation in affected areas. This might include texture discrimination tasks, where the person learns to distinguish between different materials using the affected area.

The exercises should be performed regularly but not to the point of causing severe pain. The goal is to challenge the nervous system without overwhelming it. Progress is typically gradual, with small improvements building over time.

## Case Example: Jennifer's CRPS Recovery

Jennifer, a 35-year-old office worker, developed complex regional pain syndrome (CRPS) in her right hand after a minor wrist injury. The pain was severe and burning, and her hand became extremely sensitive to touch, temperature, and movement.

Initially, Jennifer protected her hand from any stimulation, which seemed to worsen her symptoms. Her pain specialist explained that avoiding stimulation could actually maintain the hypersensitivity and recommended a desensitization program.

The desensitization program began with very gentle stimuli that Jennifer could tolerate. This included touching different textures for brief periods and gradually increasing the duration and intensity of stimulation. The process was challenging but necessary for recovery.

Jennifer also learned to use her affected hand for progressively more challenging activities. This graded motor imagery helped retrain her brain's representation of the hand while improving function. The process required significant commitment but produced gradual improvements.

After six months of consistent desensitization work, Jennifer's hand sensitivity had decreased significantly. While still present, the pain was manageable, and she could use her hand for most daily activities. Her case illustrates how desensitization can help reverse the hypersensitivity associated with neuropathic pain.

## Mirror Therapy and Graded Motor Imagery

Mirror therapy and graded motor imagery are innovative approaches that use the brain's plasticity to reduce neuropathic pain. These techniques are particularly useful for conditions like CRPS, phantom limb pain, and other forms of neuropathic pain that involve changes in brain representation.

## Mirror Therapy

Mirror therapy involves using a mirror to create the illusion that the affected limb is moving normally. The person performs exercises with the unaffected limb while watching its reflection in the mirror, creating the visual illusion that the affected limb is moving without pain.

This technique works by providing the brain with normal visual feedback about limb movement, which can help restore normal brain representation of the affected area. The treatment is typically performed for 15-30 minutes daily over several weeks or months.

Research has shown that mirror therapy can significantly reduce pain and improve function in people with CRPS, phantom limb pain, and other neuropathic conditions. The treatment is safe, inexpensive, and can be performed at home.

## Graded Motor Imagery

Graded motor imagery is a more complex approach that involves three progressive stages: laterality recognition, explicit motor imagery, and mirror therapy. Each stage is designed to gradually retrain the brain's representation of the affected area.

Laterality recognition involves identifying whether images of hands or feet are left or right. This simple task helps assess and improve the brain's representation of body parts. People with CRPS often have difficulty with this task, which improves with practice.

Explicit motor imagery involves imagining movements of the affected limb without actually moving it. This mental rehearsal helps activate brain regions involved in movement planning and may reduce pain while improving function.

## Case Example: Robert's Mirror Therapy Success

Robert, a 28-year-old mechanic, developed CRPS in his left arm after a work-related injury. The pain was constant and burning, with severe sensitivity to touch and movement. Traditional treatments had provided minimal relief, and Robert was becoming increasingly disabled by his condition.

His occupational therapist introduced mirror therapy as part of his treatment plan. Robert was initially skeptical about how looking at his reflection could help with his pain, but he was willing to try anything that might provide relief.

The mirror therapy sessions began with simple exercises using his unaffected right arm while watching its reflection in the mirror. The visual illusion created the appearance that his left arm was moving normally without pain. Initially, Robert found the exercises strange and difficult.

Over several weeks of daily practice, Robert began to notice subtle changes in his pain levels. The burning sensation in his left arm decreased, and he could tolerate light touch more easily. The visual feedback seemed to be helping his brain relearn normal movement patterns.

Robert progressed through the graded motor imagery program, adding laterality recognition exercises and explicit motor imagery. Each component contributed to his overall improvement, helping retrain his brain's representation of his affected arm.

After three months of consistent mirror therapy practice, Robert's pain had decreased by 70%. He was able to return to light work activities and had regained significant function in his left arm. His case demonstrates how innovative approaches can help people with severe neuropathic pain.

## Complex Regional Pain Syndrome

CRPS represents one of the most challenging neuropathic pain conditions, characterized by severe burning pain, swelling, and changes in skin color and temperature. The condition typically develops after an injury, but the pain and other symptoms are disproportionate to the original injury.

## CRPS Pathophysiology

CRPS involves dysfunction in both the peripheral and central nervous systems. The sympathetic nervous system, which normally regulates blood flow and sweating, becomes overactive and contributes to the pain and other symptoms.

Inflammation plays a significant role in CRPS, particularly in the early stages. The affected limb may become swollen, warm, and red, resembling an infection. However, this inflammation is neurogenic - caused by nerve dysfunction rather than infection.

Changes in brain representation of the affected limb contribute to CRPS symptoms. Brain imaging studies show that people with CRPS have altered representation of the affected limb in the somatosensory cortex, which may contribute to both pain and movement problems.

## CRPS Treatment Approaches

Early intervention is crucial for CRPS management. The condition can progress rapidly, and early treatment may prevent the development of more severe symptoms. This makes prompt diagnosis and treatment essential.

Physical therapy plays a central role in CRPS treatment, though it must be approached carefully. The goal is to maintain function and prevent contractures while avoiding activities that significantly worsen symptoms. This requires a delicate balance between activity and rest.

Sympathetic nerve blocks can provide significant relief for some people with CRPS, particularly in the early stages. These procedures involve injecting local anesthetic near sympathetic nerves to interrupt the abnormal nerve activity contributing to symptoms.

## Case Example: Sarah's CRPS Management

Sarah, a 42-year-old teacher, developed CRPS in her right foot after a minor ankle sprain. What should have been a simple injury that healed in a few weeks instead became a condition that caused severe burning pain and prevented her from walking normally.

The diagnosis of CRPS was made several months after the initial injury, when it became clear that Sarah's symptoms were disproportionate to the original injury. Her foot was hypersensitive to touch, and she experienced severe pain with any weight-bearing activities.

Sarah's treatment plan included multiple approaches to address the complex nature of CRPS. She was started on gabapentin for neuropathic pain, which provided some relief but wasn't sufficient to restore function.

Physical therapy was crucial for Sarah's recovery but required careful modification. The therapist used desensitization techniques to gradually reduce her foot's hypersensitivity while maintaining as much function as possible. Progress was slow but steady.

Sarah also received sympathetic nerve blocks, which provided temporary but significant relief. These procedures allowed her to participate more fully in physical therapy and gradually increase her activity level.

The combination of medications, physical therapy, and procedures allowed Sarah to make significant progress. After one year of intensive treatment, she was able to return to teaching and had regained most of her normal function.

## Managing Neuropathic Pain Flares

Neuropathic pain can be unpredictable, with periods of relative stability interrupted by flares of increased pain. Having strategies for managing these flares is essential for maintaining quality of life and preventing the development of fear-avoidance behaviors.

**Flare Prevention Strategies**

Identifying triggers that precipitate neuropathic pain flares can help prevent them. Common triggers include stress, weather changes, lack of sleep, and certain activities. Keeping a pain diary can help identify personal triggers.

Maintaining consistent medication schedules helps prevent fluctuations in pain levels. Skipping doses or taking medications irregularly can lead to breakthrough pain and increased sensitivity.

Stress management is particularly important for neuropathic pain because stress can directly worsen nerve sensitivity. Regular practice of relaxation techniques, exercise, and other stress-reduction strategies can help prevent flares.

**Acute Flare Management**

Having a plan for managing acute flares helps prevent panic and ensures appropriate treatment. This might include rescue medications, specific positioning techniques, or relaxation strategies that have been effective in the past.

Topical treatments can provide localized relief during flares. Ice or heat (depending on individual response), topical analgesics, or prescribed topical medications can help manage acute increases in pain.

Activity modification during flares is important but should be balanced with maintaining function. Complete rest may worsen symptoms, while excessive activity can prolong flares. The key is finding the right balance for each individual.

**Case Example: Michael's Flare Management System**

Michael, a 55-year-old accountant with diabetic neuropathy, experienced unpredictable flares that would dramatically increase his foot pain for days at a time. These flares were disrupting his work and causing significant anxiety about when the next episode would occur.

Michael worked with his physician to develop a comprehensive flare management plan. This included identifying his personal triggers, which included stress at work, changes in weather, and disruptions to his sleep schedule.

The plan included both preventive and acute management strategies. Michael learned stress management techniques and worked to maintain consistent sleep patterns. He also ensured his diabetes was well-controlled, which helped reduce the frequency of flares.

For acute flares, Michael had a specific protocol that included adjusting his medication dosing (under medical supervision), using topical treatments, and modifying his activities. Having this plan reduced his anxiety and helped him manage flares more effectively.

Michael also learned to recognize early warning signs of flares, which allowed him to implement interventions before the pain became severe. This proactive approach helped reduce both the frequency and severity of his flares.

## Building Your Neuropathic Pain Management Team

Neuropathic pain is complex and often requires input from multiple healthcare providers. Each team member brings specialized knowledge and skills that contribute to optimal outcomes.

## Pain Management Specialists

Pain management specialists have expertise in the complex mechanisms of neuropathic pain and access to specialized treatments. They can provide interventional procedures, complex medication management, and coordination of care.

## Neurologists

Neurologists can help diagnose the underlying causes of neuropathic pain and provide treatments for specific neurological conditions. They're particularly important for conditions like trigeminal neuralgia, which may require specialized treatments.

## Physical and Occupational Therapists

Physical therapists can design exercise programs that maintain function while managing pain. They're skilled in techniques like desensitization and graded exposure that are particularly important for neuropathic pain conditions.

Occupational therapists focus on daily activities and can recommend adaptive equipment and techniques that reduce pain while maintaining independence. They're particularly helpful for people with hand and arm neuropathic pain.

### Mental Health Professionals

Neuropathic pain can significantly impact mental health, and addressing psychological factors is often essential for optimal outcomes. Mental health professionals can provide counseling, stress management techniques, and treatment for depression and anxiety.

### The Path Forward

Neuropathic pain management continues to evolve with new understanding of pain mechanisms and the development of targeted treatments. While these conditions can be challenging, many people are able to achieve significant improvement with appropriate treatment.

Success in neuropathic pain management often requires patience and persistence. The treatments may take time to work, and finding the right combination of approaches may require trial and adjustment. However, the potential for meaningful improvement exists for most people.

The final chapters of this book will integrate the information from previous chapters into practical treatment planning approaches that can help you develop a comprehensive pain management strategy.

### Nerve Pain Navigation

Neuropathic pain presents unique challenges that require specialized approaches different from other types of pain. Understanding the mechanisms involved helps explain why traditional pain treatments often fail and why targeted therapies are necessary.

The key to successful neuropathic pain management lies in early intervention, appropriate medication selection, and the integration of multiple treatment approaches. While these conditions can be challenging, significant improvement is possible with proper treatment.

**Neuropathic Pain Management Principles:**

- Neuropathic pain arises from nerve dysfunction rather than tissue damage, requiring specialized treatments

- First-line treatments include gabapentinoids, certain antidepressants, and topical medications

- Desensitization techniques can help reduce hypersensitivity and improve function

- Mirror therapy and graded motor imagery utilize brain plasticity to reduce pain

- CRPS requires early, intensive intervention to prevent progression and disability

- Flare management strategies help maintain quality of life during symptom exacerbations

# Chapter 15: Creating Your Personal Pain Management Plan

The most sophisticated pain management approaches in the world are worthless if they don't work for your specific situation. This chapter brings together all the previous information into a practical framework you can use to develop your own personalized pain management strategy. The key isn't finding the "perfect" plan - it's creating a systematic approach that you can modify and improve over time.

Think of this process as building a house. You need a solid foundation (assessment and goal setting), a clear blueprint (combining modalities), and regular inspections (tracking progress) to ensure everything is working as intended. Just as a house needs occasional renovations and updates, your pain management plan will need adjustments as your condition changes and new treatments become available.

## Assessment Tools for Pain and Function

Effective pain management begins with accurate assessment. You can't manage what you don't measure, and subjective pain experiences need to be quantified to track progress and guide treatment decisions. The challenge lies in translating your personal pain experience into measurable data that can inform treatment choices.

## Pain Rating Scales

The numeric rating scale (0-10) is the most commonly used pain assessment tool, but it's often used incorrectly. Many people think of 10 as "the worst pain I've ever experienced," but this creates a moving target that changes as you experience different pain levels. Instead, 10 should represent "the worst pain imaginable" - a theoretical maximum that remains constant.

The scale should also account for different dimensions of pain. A 6/10 sharp, stabbing pain feels different from a 6/10 dull, aching pain. Consider rating both intensity and quality separately to provide more complete information about your pain experience.

Functional pain scales can be more useful than simple intensity ratings. These scales describe how pain affects your daily activities: 0 means no pain, 5 means pain that interferes with some activities, and 10 means pain that prevents all activities. This approach connects pain ratings to real-world impacts.

## Functional Assessment Tools

The Pain Disability Index (PDI) measures how pain affects seven life areas: family responsibilities, recreation, social activities, occupation, sexual behavior, self-care, and life-support activities. Each area is rated from 0 (no disability) to 10 (total disability), providing a comprehensive picture of pain's impact.

The Oswestry Disability Index specifically assesses how back pain affects daily activities like lifting, walking, sitting, and sleeping. This tool is particularly useful for people with spinal conditions because it focuses on activities commonly affected by back pain.

Activity-specific assessments can be more relevant than general functional measures. If your pain primarily affects your ability to work, cook, or exercise, create personalized assessments that focus on these specific activities.

## Case Example: Margaret's Assessment Evolution

Margaret, a 51-year-old teacher with fibromyalgia, initially rated her pain as "bad" or "really bad" without providing useful information for treatment planning. Her physician introduced structured assessment tools that helped quantify her pain experience and track treatment progress.

Margaret began using a pain diary that included not just intensity ratings but also pain quality, location, triggers, and functional impact. She rated her pain intensity on a 0-10 scale while also noting descriptors like "burning," "aching," or "stabbing" to capture pain quality.

The functional assessment revealed that Margaret's pain most significantly affected her sleep quality and energy levels. While her pain intensity might rate 6/10, her fatigue and sleep disruption were more disabling than the pain itself. This information helped guide treatment priorities.

Margaret also tracked her activity levels and mood alongside her pain ratings. She discovered that her pain intensity didn't always correlate with her function - some days she felt worse but could still accomplish daily tasks, while other days moderate pain was completely disabling.

After six months of structured assessment, Margaret and her healthcare team had a clear picture of her pain patterns and functional limitations. This information guided treatment decisions and helped track progress more effectively than simple pain ratings alone.

The assessment tools helped Margaret become more aware of her pain patterns and triggers. She learned to recognize early warning signs of flares and could implement interventions before symptoms became severe. This proactive approach improved her overall pain management.

### Goal Setting for Pain Management

Effective goal setting in pain management requires balancing optimism with realism. The goal isn't to eliminate all pain - that's unrealistic for most chronic conditions - but to reduce pain to manageable levels while improving function and quality of life.

### SMART Goals Framework

SMART goals are Specific, Measurable, Achievable, Relevant, and Time-bound. Instead of "I want to feel better," a SMART goal might be "I will reduce my average daily pain from 7/10 to 5/10 within three months by implementing a daily exercise routine and stress management techniques."

Specific goals focus on particular aspects of pain management. Rather than general improvement, target specific activities like "I will be able to walk for 20 minutes without stopping" or "I will sleep through the night at least five nights per week."

Measurable goals use quantifiable metrics to track progress. This might include pain intensity ratings, functional assessments, medication usage, or activity levels. The key is having objective measures that can be tracked over time.

Achievable goals are realistic given your current condition and resources. Setting overly ambitious goals leads to frustration and abandonment of the plan. Start with modest goals and build on success rather than attempting dramatic changes.

Relevant goals address the aspects of pain that most impact your life. If work performance is your primary concern, focus on goals that improve your ability to function professionally. If family activities are most important, prioritize goals that support those activities.

Time-bound goals have specific deadlines that create accountability and urgency. Without deadlines, goals become wishes rather than actionable plans. Set both short-term (weekly/monthly) and long-term (3-6 months) goals.

**Functional vs. Pain-Focused Goals**

Functional goals often produce better outcomes than pain-focused goals because they address what matters most to you. Instead of "reduce pain by 50%," consider "return to playing with my grandchildren" or "complete a full day of work without pain interfering."

Activity-based goals provide clear targets for improvement. "I will walk for 30 minutes daily" is more actionable than "I will improve my fitness." These goals also provide natural progression paths as you build capacity.

Quality of life goals address broader impacts of pain management. This might include social activities, hobbies, or personal relationships that have been affected by pain. These goals help maintain motivation by connecting pain management to meaningful life activities.

**Case Example: David's Goal-Setting Success**

David, a 46-year-old carpenter with chronic back pain, initially set the goal of "getting rid of my back pain completely." This unrealistic goal led to frustration when treatments didn't provide complete relief, causing him to abandon several potentially helpful approaches.

His physical therapist helped David reframe his goals using the SMART framework. Instead of eliminating pain, David focused on functional improvements that would allow him to return to work and maintain his active lifestyle.

David's primary goal became "return to work as a carpenter within six months while maintaining pain levels below 6/10." This goal was specific, measurable, and relevant to his priorities. He also set supporting goals around exercise, sleep, and stress management.

The goal-setting process helped David identify what aspects of his condition were most important to address. He realized that morning stiffness and fatigue were often more limiting than pain intensity, leading to treatment adjustments that addressed these specific issues.

David broke his main goal into smaller, achievable steps. He started with "work for two hours without increased pain," then progressed to "complete a half-day of light carpentry work." Each success built confidence and motivation to continue.

After eight months, David had achieved his goal of returning to work, though with some modifications to his activities. His pain levels were manageable, and he felt confident in his ability to maintain his improvements long-term.

## Combining Modalities for Maximum Effect

The real power of pain management comes from combining different approaches that work together to address multiple aspects of your pain experience. Research published in ScienceDirect has documented the benefits of multimodal approaches, showing that combinations of treatments often produce better outcomes than any single intervention alone (90).

## Understanding Treatment Interactions

Some treatments work better together than separately. Physical therapy combined with stress management techniques can address both physical and psychological aspects of pain. Medications can make exercise more tolerable, while exercise can reduce medication requirements.

Timing matters when combining treatments. Taking pain medication before physical therapy might allow for better participation, while relaxation techniques before sleep can improve rest quality. Understanding these interactions helps optimize your treatment plan.

Some combinations should be avoided or used carefully. Combining multiple sedating medications can cause excessive drowsiness, while certain supplements can interact with prescription drugs. Always discuss combination approaches with your healthcare providers.

## Building Your Treatment Stack

Start with foundational treatments that address the most significant aspects of your pain. This might include movement therapy for physical conditioning, sleep hygiene for restorative rest, and stress management for emotional well-being.

Add targeted treatments that address specific symptoms or limitations. If muscle tension is a major issue, consider massage therapy or heat applications. If mood is significantly affected, psychological support might be beneficial.

Advanced treatments like neuromodulation or specialized procedures should be considered after foundational approaches are established. These treatments work best when combined with good self-management skills and healthy lifestyle habits.

## Case Example: Lisa's Multimodal Approach

Lisa, a 41-year-old office manager with chronic neck pain, initially tried one treatment at a time without success. Physical therapy helped temporarily, but benefits didn't last. Medications provided some relief but caused side effects that limited their usefulness.

Lisa's pain management team recommended a multimodal approach that combined several treatments simultaneously. The plan included physical therapy, stress management training, ergonomic workplace modifications, and targeted medications.

The physical therapy addressed muscle imbalances and movement dysfunction that contributed to Lisa's neck pain. Stress management techniques helped her cope with work pressures that seemed to worsen her symptoms. Workplace modifications reduced repetitive strain.

The treatments worked together in ways that enhanced each other's effectiveness. Stress management made physical therapy more tolerable, while improved physical conditioning reduced her stress levels. Workplace modifications reduced the triggers that caused flares.

Lisa also learned to adjust her treatment approach based on her symptoms and life circumstances. During busy periods at work, she increased her stress management practices. When her pain was higher, she focused more on physical treatments.

After one year of multimodal treatment, Lisa had achieved significant improvements in both pain levels and function. She understood how different treatments worked together and felt confident in her ability to manage her condition long-term.

## Tracking Progress Through Technology and Traditional Methods

Consistent tracking provides the feedback necessary to optimize your pain management plan. Without objective measures of progress, it's easy to lose motivation or continue ineffective treatments. The key is finding tracking methods that provide useful information without becoming burdensome.

### Digital Pain Tracking

Smartphone apps offer convenient ways to track pain patterns, medication use, and treatment effectiveness. Many apps include features like weather tracking, mood monitoring, and activity logging that can help identify triggers and patterns.

The key to successful digital tracking is consistency. Choose an app that's easy to use and provides the information you need without excessive complexity. Simple interfaces with quick data entry work better than complex systems that require significant time investment.

Look for apps that allow data export or sharing with healthcare providers. This feature enables your medical team to review your tracking data and make informed treatment decisions based on objective information.

### Traditional Tracking Methods

Paper diaries remain effective for people who prefer traditional methods or have limited technology access. The advantage of paper tracking is that it forces you to actively consider your pain and treatment response.

Weekly summaries can capture trends that daily tracking might miss. Instead of rating pain every day, consider weekly averages and patterns. This approach reduces tracking burden while providing useful information.

Monthly reviews allow for broader pattern recognition and treatment evaluation. Set aside time each month to review your tracking data and identify trends, successes, and areas for improvement.

**Case Example: Robert's Tracking Transformation**

Robert, a 58-year-old with arthritis, initially dismissed pain tracking as "too much work." His physician convinced him to try a simple smartphone app for one month to see if it provided useful information.

The app revealed patterns that Robert hadn't noticed. His pain was consistently worse on Mondays and Tuesdays, which correlated with weekend activities that involved more physical work around his house. This information helped him adjust his activity pacing.

Robert also discovered that his pain levels were influenced by weather changes, particularly drops in barometric pressure. While he couldn't control the weather, knowing this trigger helped him prepare for potential flares with appropriate medications and activity modifications.

The tracking data helped Robert's healthcare team make informed treatment decisions. They could see which medications were most effective and adjust dosing based on his pain patterns rather than relying on his recall of symptoms.

After six months of tracking, Robert had a clear picture of his pain patterns and treatment responses. This information guided modifications to his treatment plan that resulted in better pain control and improved function.

**Adjusting Your Approach Based on Results**

Pain management plans require regular adjustment based on results, changing circumstances, and new treatment options. The International Association for the Study of Pain has published guidelines on pain management that emphasize the importance of ongoing assessment and plan modification (91, 92, 93, 94, 95, 96, 97, 98, 99).

## Recognizing When Changes Are Needed

Treatment plateaus occur when initial improvements level off or stop. This is normal and doesn't necessarily mean the treatment isn't working. However, it may indicate the need for plan modifications or additional treatments.

Worsening symptoms despite treatment compliance suggest the need for plan revision. This might involve increasing treatment intensity, adding new modalities, or addressing previously unidentified factors contributing to pain.

Life changes can necessitate plan adjustments. New job demands, family responsibilities, or health conditions may require modifications to your pain management approach. The plan should adapt to your changing circumstances.

## Making Systematic Adjustments

Change one variable at a time to identify what's helping and what isn't. Making multiple changes simultaneously makes it impossible to determine which modifications are beneficial.

Give changes adequate time to work before making additional adjustments. Most treatments require several weeks or months to show their full effects. Premature changes can disrupt potentially beneficial treatments.

Document all changes and their effects to learn what works best for your specific situation. This information becomes valuable for future treatment decisions and helps avoid repeating unsuccessful approaches.

## Case Example: Jennifer's Plan Evolution

Jennifer, a 44-year-old nurse with fibromyalgia, developed a comprehensive pain management plan that worked well for two years. However, a job change to a more stressful position led to increased symptoms that her existing plan couldn't manage.

Jennifer's healthcare team reviewed her tracking data and identified that stress was the primary factor in her symptom increase. They modified her plan to include additional stress management techniques and adjusted her medication regimen.

The plan modifications included mindfulness training, workplace stress reduction strategies, and a temporary increase in her sleep medication. These changes addressed the specific factors that were worsening her symptoms.

Jennifer also learned to recognize early signs of stress-related symptom increases. She developed strategies for managing work stress proactively rather than waiting for symptoms to worsen before taking action.

After three months of plan modifications, Jennifer's symptoms had returned to manageable levels. She had developed skills for managing stress-related flares and felt confident in her ability to adapt her plan as needed.

## Building Long-Term Success

Creating a sustainable pain management plan requires thinking beyond immediate symptom relief to long-term health and function. The most effective plans are those that can be maintained and modified over time as your needs change.

## Sustainability Factors

Choose treatments that fit your lifestyle and preferences. The best treatment plan is one you'll actually follow consistently. Consider your schedule, resources, and personal preferences when selecting approaches.

Build flexibility into your plan to accommodate changing circumstances. Life events, seasonal changes, and evolving symptoms all require plan adjustments. A rigid plan that can't be modified is likely to fail.

Develop problem-solving skills for managing setbacks and flares. These events are normal parts of chronic pain management, and having strategies for handling them prevents them from derailing your overall progress.

## Creating Your Personal Framework

Develop a systematic approach to pain management that includes assessment, goal setting, treatment selection, tracking, and adjustment. This framework provides structure while allowing for personalization based on your specific needs.

The framework should be simple enough to understand and implement but flexible enough to accommodate different treatments and changing circumstances. Think of it as a template that guides your decisions rather than a rigid protocol.

Regular review and update of your framework ensures it remains relevant and effective. Schedule monthly or quarterly reviews to assess progress and make necessary adjustments.

## Moving Forward with Confidence

The next chapter will focus on building effective relationships with healthcare providers, an essential component of successful pain management. You'll learn how to communicate effectively, advocate for your needs, and build a healthcare team that supports your goals.

## Personal Pain Management Mastery

Creating a personal pain management plan is both an art and a science. It requires systematic assessment, realistic goal setting, and the wisdom to combine treatments in ways that address your unique situation. The process takes time and patience, but the results can be transformative.

Success comes from understanding that pain management is a journey rather than a destination. Your plan will evolve as you learn what works, as your condition changes, and as new treatments become available. The key is maintaining a systematic approach while remaining flexible enough to adapt to changing circumstances.

**Planning and Progress Principles:**

- Structured assessment tools provide objective measures of pain and function

- SMART goals create clear targets for improvement while maintaining realistic expectations

- Multimodal approaches combining different treatments often produce better outcomes than single interventions

- Consistent tracking provides feedback necessary for plan optimization and motivation

- Regular plan adjustments based on results and changing circumstances ensure continued effectiveness

- Sustainable plans that fit your lifestyle and preferences are more likely to succeed long-term

# Chapter 16: Working with Healthcare Providers

Healthcare is fundamentally a team sport, yet many people with chronic pain feel isolated and frustrated in their interactions with medical professionals. The complexity of pain management requires coordination between multiple providers, each bringing specialized knowledge and skills to your care. Success depends not just on finding the right providers but on building productive relationships that support your goals.

The challenge lies in bridging the gap between your lived experience of pain and the clinical approach that healthcare providers use to assess and treat conditions. You experience pain as a complex, personal phenomenon that affects every aspect of your life. Providers see pain through the lens of medical training, diagnostic criteria, and treatment algorithms. Effective communication requires translating between these different perspectives.

**Building Your Pain Management Team**

The composition of your healthcare team depends on your specific condition, treatment needs, and available resources. However, most successful pain management approaches involve coordination between multiple providers who understand their roles and communicate effectively with each other.

**Primary Care as Your Foundation**

Your primary care physician serves as the quarterback of your pain management team. They coordinate care, manage overall health, and provide continuity when you're working with multiple specialists. A good primary care relationship is essential for effective pain management.

Primary care providers can handle many aspects of pain management, including basic medications, lifestyle counseling, and referrals to specialists. They also monitor for complications and ensure that pain management doesn't interfere with other aspects of your health.

The key is finding a primary care provider who understands pain management and is willing to coordinate with specialists. Not all primary care providers are comfortable managing complex pain conditions, so it's important to find one who shares your treatment philosophy and goals.

### Specialist Roles and Referrals

Pain management specialists have advanced training in complex pain conditions and access to specialized treatments. They can provide interventional procedures, complex medication management, and expertise in difficult cases.

Rheumatologists specialize in inflammatory conditions like arthritis and can provide expert diagnosis and treatment for these conditions. They're particularly important for autoimmune conditions that require specialized medications.

Neurologists focus on nervous system conditions and can be helpful for neuropathic pain, headaches, and other neurological causes of pain. They have expertise in brain and nerve function that can be crucial for certain conditions.

Physical medicine and rehabilitation (PM&R) physicians specialize in restoring function and improving quality of life. They often serve as pain management specialists with additional expertise in rehabilitation approaches.

### Case Example: Maria's Team Building Success

Maria, a 45-year-old teacher with rheumatoid arthritis, initially tried to manage her condition through her primary care physician alone. While well-intentioned, her doctor lacked the specialized knowledge needed to optimize her treatment.

Maria's symptoms worsened despite basic treatment, leading to significant disability and work limitations. Her primary care physician recognized the need for specialized care and referred her to a rheumatologist.

The rheumatologist provided expert diagnosis and treatment with disease-modifying medications that her primary care physician wasn't comfortable prescribing. The specialized care led to significant improvement in Maria's symptoms and function.

However, Maria discovered that specialized care alone wasn't sufficient. She needed physical therapy for exercise guidance, occupational therapy for workplace modifications, and psychological support for coping with chronic illness.

Building her team required coordination between providers. Maria's primary care physician served as the central coordinator, while the rheumatologist provided specialized medical management. The therapists addressed specific functional needs.

The team approach provided Maria with comprehensive care that addressed all aspects of her condition. Each provider contributed their expertise while working toward shared goals. This coordination led to better outcomes than any single provider could have achieved alone.

**Mental Health Integration**

Chronic pain significantly impacts mental health, and addressing psychological factors is often essential for optimal outcomes. This doesn't mean your pain is psychological - it means that pain affects your emotions, thoughts, and behaviors in ways that can be addressed therapeutically.

Pain psychologists specialize in the psychological aspects of chronic pain and can provide cognitive behavioral therapy, stress management training, and coping skills. They understand the unique challenges of living with chronic pain.

Psychiatrists can prescribe medications for depression, anxiety, and other mental health conditions that often accompany chronic pain. Some antidepressants also have direct pain-relieving effects.

**Case Example: Robert's Mental Health Integration**

Robert, a 52-year-old construction worker with chronic back pain, initially resisted suggestions about psychological support. He felt that this implied his pain wasn't real or that he was "weak" for needing help.

Robert's pain management specialist explained that chronic pain affects brain chemistry and that psychological support could help him develop better coping skills. The focus wasn't on whether his pain was real but on how to manage its impact on his life.

Robert agreed to try a few sessions with a pain psychologist. The therapist helped him understand the connection between his thoughts, emotions, and pain experience. Robert learned that his catastrophic thinking was actually increasing his pain levels.

The psychological support helped Robert develop better coping strategies and reduce the emotional distress that was amplifying his pain. He learned relaxation techniques and strategies for managing pain flares.

Robert's pain levels decreased significantly once he addressed the psychological factors that were contributing to his suffering. He realized that getting psychological support was actually a sign of strength rather than weakness.

**Effective Communication with Healthcare Providers**

Clear communication between you and your healthcare providers is essential for effective pain management. Yet many people struggle to convey their pain experience in ways that providers can understand and act upon. The key is learning to translate your subjective experience into objective information that guides treatment decisions.

**Preparing for Appointments**

Come prepared with specific information about your pain patterns, triggers, and treatment responses. Vague descriptions like "I hurt all over" are less helpful than specific details about location, intensity, and timing.

Keep a pain diary for at least two weeks before appointments to provide objective data about your symptoms. Include information about what makes your pain better or worse, how it affects your daily activities, and any patterns you've noticed.

Research published in Oxford Academic and Psychology Today has shown that patients who prepare for appointments and communicate effectively with their healthcare providers achieve better outcomes (100, 101).

Bring a list of questions and concerns to ensure you don't forget important topics during the appointment. Prioritize your questions so that the most important issues are addressed first.

**Describing Your Pain Effectively**

Use specific descriptors for your pain quality. Words like "burning," "stabbing," "throbbing," or "electric" provide more information than "bad" or "severe." These descriptors help providers understand the type of pain you're experiencing.

Quantify your pain using the 0-10 scale consistently. Remember that 0 means no pain and 10 means the worst pain imaginable. Use the same reference point each time to ensure your ratings are comparable.

Describe how pain affects your function rather than just its intensity. "I can't sleep because of pain" or "I can't lift my grandchildren" provides more useful information than pain intensity ratings alone.

**Case Example: Linda's Communication Breakthrough**

Linda, a 38-year-old office worker with chronic headaches, initially struggled to communicate effectively with her healthcare providers. She would describe her pain as "really bad" or "terrible" without providing specific information that could guide treatment.

Linda's physician taught her to use more specific descriptors and to track her headache patterns. She learned to describe her pain as "throbbing on the left side" or "pressure around both temples" rather than just "headache."

The improved communication led to better treatment decisions. Her physician could distinguish between different types of headaches and tailor treatments accordingly. Linda's headache frequency decreased significantly once she received appropriate treatment.

Linda also learned to advocate for herself when treatments weren't working. Instead of suffering in silence, she would call her physician's office to report problems and request adjustments to her treatment plan.

The communication skills Linda developed improved all her healthcare interactions. She felt more confident discussing her symptoms and more satisfied with the care she received.

### Navigating Insurance Coverage

Insurance coverage for pain management services can be complex and varies significantly between plans. Understanding your benefits and advocating for necessary treatments is an important part of effective pain management.

### Understanding Your Benefits

Review your insurance policy to understand what pain management services are covered. This includes medications, procedures, therapy services, and specialist visits. Know your copays, deductibles, and any preauthorization requirements.

Many insurance plans have different coverage levels for different types of providers. Physical therapy might be covered differently than massage therapy, and pain management procedures might require special approval.

Alternative treatments like acupuncture, chiropractic care, and massage therapy have varying coverage depending on your plan.

Some plans cover these services while others don't, so it's important to understand your specific benefits.

## Advocating for Coverage

If a treatment is denied, you have the right to appeal the decision. Work with your healthcare provider to provide medical justification for the treatment and documentation of its necessity.

Prior authorization requirements can delay treatment but are often necessary for specialized procedures or medications. Your healthcare provider's office should help navigate these requirements.

Document all communications with your insurance company, including claim numbers, representative names, and dates of calls. This documentation can be helpful if disputes arise.

## Case Example: David's Insurance Navigation

David, a 47-year-old with complex regional pain syndrome, needed specialized treatments that his insurance company initially denied. The treatments were expensive, and David couldn't afford them without insurance coverage.

David's pain management physician provided detailed medical justification for the treatments, including research evidence and documentation of failed alternative treatments. This information supported the medical necessity of the proposed treatments.

The insurance company initially denied the treatments, but David appealed the decision with his physician's support. The appeal process took several weeks but ultimately resulted in approval for the necessary treatments.

David learned to work proactively with his insurance company rather than waiting for denials. He would call to verify coverage before scheduling treatments and ensure that prior authorizations were in place.

The insurance navigation skills David developed helped him access the treatments he needed while minimizing out-of-pocket costs. He became an effective advocate for his own care.

## When to Consider Specialist Referrals

Knowing when to seek specialized care can significantly impact your pain management outcomes. While primary care providers can manage many pain conditions, certain situations require specialized expertise.

## Indications for Specialist Referral

Persistent pain that doesn't respond to basic treatments may require specialized evaluation. If you've tried multiple approaches without success, a specialist might identify underlying factors that haven't been addressed.

Complex conditions like CRPS, fibromyalgia, or autoimmune disorders often require specialized expertise for optimal management. These conditions have specific treatment approaches that general practitioners may not be familiar with.

The need for specialized procedures or medications that primary care providers aren't comfortable managing is another indication for referral. This might include injections, nerve blocks, or complex medication regimens.

## Choosing the Right Specialist

Research potential specialists before making appointments. Look for board certification in relevant specialties and experience treating your specific condition. Online reviews and referrals from other patients can provide useful information.

Consider the specialist's treatment philosophy and approach. Some specialists focus primarily on medications, while others emphasize multidisciplinary approaches. Choose someone whose approach aligns with your preferences and goals.

Location and accessibility are practical considerations that affect your ability to maintain ongoing care. Specialists who are too far away or difficult to schedule with may not be practical choices for long-term care.

**Case Example: Jennifer's Specialist Journey**

Jennifer, a 41-year-old with fibromyalgia, spent months trying to get effective treatment from her primary care physician. While well-meaning, her doctor lacked the specialized knowledge needed to manage her complex condition.

Jennifer's symptoms continued to worsen despite basic treatments, leading to significant disability and quality of life impacts. Her primary care physician finally referred her to a rheumatologist who specialized in fibromyalgia.

The rheumatologist provided a comprehensive evaluation that identified several factors contributing to Jennifer's symptoms. The specialist had access to medications and treatment approaches that weren't available through primary care.

Jennifer's treatment plan included specialized medications, referrals to appropriate therapists, and education about fibromyalgia management. The coordinated approach led to significant improvement in her symptoms and function.

The specialist also provided ongoing support and adjustment of her treatment plan as needed. This specialized care was essential for managing Jennifer's complex condition effectively.

**Advocating for Your Healthcare Rights**

Effective self-advocacy is essential for getting the care you need and deserve. This involves understanding your rights as a patient, communicating effectively with providers, and being persistent when necessary.

## Patient Rights and Responsibilities

You have the right to receive appropriate medical care for your pain condition. This includes access to effective treatments, adequate pain assessment, and referrals to specialists when needed.

You also have the right to be treated with dignity and respect, regardless of your pain condition. Stigma and discrimination against people with chronic pain are unfortunately common but are not acceptable.

Your responsibilities include being honest about your symptoms, following treatment recommendations, and communicating openly with your healthcare providers. Partnership works better than adversarial relationships.

## Effective Self-Advocacy Strategies

Be persistent but respectful when advocating for your needs. If one approach doesn't work, try different strategies or consider seeking care elsewhere. Don't give up if your first attempts aren't successful.

Bring support people to appointments when possible. A friend or family member can help you remember important information and provide emotional support during difficult discussions.

Document your healthcare experiences, including appointment dates, treatments tried, and outcomes. This information can be valuable when seeking care from new providers or appealing insurance decisions.

## Case Example: Michael's Advocacy Success

Michael, a 55-year-old with chronic pain, initially accepted whatever treatment his physicians recommended without question. This passive approach led to inadequate pain management and continued suffering.

Michael learned to research his condition and treatment options, which helped him have more informed discussions with his healthcare providers. He began asking questions about alternative treatments and requesting referrals when appropriate.

When one physician dismissed his concerns about medication side effects, Michael sought a second opinion. The new physician was more responsive to his concerns and helped him find a better treatment approach.

Michael's advocacy skills improved over time, and he became more confident in his interactions with healthcare providers. He learned to balance respect for medical expertise with advocacy for his own needs.

The advocacy skills Michael developed led to better healthcare outcomes and improved quality of life. He felt more in control of his healthcare and more satisfied with the care he received.

## Building Long-Term Healthcare Relationships

Chronic pain management is a marathon, not a sprint. Building strong, long-term relationships with healthcare providers can significantly improve your outcomes and quality of care over time.

## Maintaining Provider Relationships

Regular communication with your healthcare providers helps maintain strong relationships and ensures continuity of care. This includes keeping appointments, following treatment recommendations, and providing feedback about outcomes.

Show appreciation for good care when you receive it. Healthcare providers are more likely to go above and beyond for patients who are respectful and appreciative of their efforts.

Be patient with the healthcare system's limitations while advocating for your needs. Understanding that providers face constraints like time pressures and insurance restrictions can help you work more effectively within the system.

## Preparing for Provider Changes

Healthcare providers sometimes leave practices or change locations, requiring you to establish new relationships. Maintain complete medical records and treatment histories to facilitate transitions to new providers.

When changing providers, request that your medical records be transferred to ensure continuity of care. This includes test results, treatment histories, and documentation of what has and hasn't worked for you.

Use provider changes as opportunities to reassess your care and consider new approaches. A fresh perspective might identify treatment options that weren't previously considered.

**Healthcare Partnership Success**

The next chapter will explore how to integrate pain management principles into your daily life, creating routines and habits that support your long-term health and well-being.

**Building Your Healthcare Foundation**

Working effectively with healthcare providers requires both communication skills and strategic thinking. The goal is to build partnerships that support your pain management goals while respecting the expertise and constraints of the healthcare system.

Success in healthcare relationships comes from understanding that you and your providers are working toward the same goal - reducing your pain and improving your quality of life. When communication breaks down or relationships become adversarial, everyone loses. The key is finding providers who share your treatment philosophy and working together to achieve your goals.

**Healthcare Collaboration Essentials:**

- Effective pain management requires coordination between multiple healthcare providers

- Clear communication about symptoms, goals, and treatment responses improves outcomes

- Insurance navigation skills help ensure access to necessary treatments

- Knowing when to seek specialist care can significantly impact treatment success

- Self-advocacy skills are essential for getting appropriate care and treatment

- Long-term provider relationships support continuity of care and better outcomes

# Chapter 17: Holistic Pain Relief Through Daily Life

Your daily routine is either your greatest ally or your worst enemy in pain management. The small decisions you make throughout each day - how you start your morning, how you structure your work, how you prepare for sleep - accumulate into powerful forces that either support healing or perpetuate suffering. This chapter shows you how to weave pain management principles into the fabric of your daily life.

The beauty of lifestyle-based pain management lies in its accessibility and sustainability. You don't need expensive equipment, complex procedures, or frequent medical appointments. Instead, you need knowledge about how daily choices affect your pain and the commitment to make changes that support your long-term health.

## Morning Routines That Set You Up for Success

How you start your day influences your pain levels, energy, and overall well-being for the next 16 hours. Many people with chronic pain dread mornings because stiffness and discomfort are often worst upon waking. However, a well-designed morning routine can transform this challenging time into a foundation for better days.

## The Science of Morning Pain

Morning stiffness occurs because your body produces less cortisol during sleep, reducing its natural anti-inflammatory effects. Additionally, prolonged immobility during sleep can cause joints to stiffen and muscles to tighten. Understanding these mechanisms helps you design countermeasures.

Your circadian rhythm also influences pain sensitivity, with pain typically feeling worse in the early morning hours. This isn't just perception - research shows that pain thresholds are actually lower in the morning, making discomfort feel more intense.

## Creating Your Pain-Smart Morning Routine

Start with gentle movement before getting out of bed. Simple stretches, ankle circles, and knee bends can help reduce stiffness and prepare your body for the day ahead. These movements stimulate circulation and begin the process of loosening tight muscles and joints.

Heat therapy can be particularly beneficial in the morning. A warm shower, heating pad, or hot compress applied to stiff areas can provide immediate relief and make movement easier. The heat increases blood flow and relaxes muscles that have tightened overnight.

Hydration is crucial after hours without fluid intake. Dehydration can increase pain sensitivity and worsen stiffness. Drink a full glass of water upon waking, and consider adding electrolytes if you tend to sweat during sleep.

**Case Example: Sarah's Morning Transformation**

Sarah, a 52-year-old with rheumatoid arthritis, used to wake up in severe pain and stiffness that made getting out of bed a 30-minute ordeal. She would lie in bed dreading the day ahead, which often started with tears of frustration and pain.

Sarah's rheumatologist suggested developing a structured morning routine that addressed her specific symptoms. The routine began before she even got out of bed, with gentle joint movements and stretches that could be done lying down.

Sarah invested in a heated mattress pad that she could turn on from her bedside table. She would wake up to gentle warmth that helped relax her stiff joints. This simple change reduced her morning pain by about 40% and made getting out of bed much easier.

The routine included a warm shower with gentle stretching under the warm water. Sarah found that the combination of heat and movement was more effective than either alone. She also used this time for deep breathing exercises that helped her start the day with a calm mindset.

Sarah's morning routine also included taking her arthritis medication with a substantial breakfast. This timing helped maximize the medication's effectiveness while minimizing stomach upset. She learned that consistency in timing was as important as the medication itself.

After implementing her morning routine, Sarah's overall pain levels decreased, and she felt more optimistic about facing each day. The routine took about 45 minutes but saved her hours of discomfort and gave her a sense of control over her condition.

### Nutrition in Your Morning Routine

What you eat in the morning can significantly impact your pain levels throughout the day. Anti-inflammatory foods like berries, nuts, and fish can help reduce systemic inflammation, while pro-inflammatory foods like processed meats and refined sugars can worsen pain.

Protein at breakfast helps stabilize blood sugar levels, which can affect pain sensitivity. Unstable blood sugar can increase inflammation and worsen pain, making protein an important component of a pain-smart breakfast.

Timing matters as much as food choices. Eating at consistent times helps regulate your body's natural rhythms and can improve the effectiveness of medications that need to be taken with food.

### Movement Integration

Gentle exercise in the morning can help reduce stiffness and improve function throughout the day. This doesn't need to be intense - simple stretching, walking, or yoga can provide significant benefits.

The key is finding activities that feel good and are sustainable. If morning exercise feels like punishment, you're less likely to maintain the routine. Start with activities you enjoy and gradually build intensity as your body adapts.

Consider your personal preferences and limitations when designing morning movement. Some people prefer gentle yoga, while others benefit from a brisk walk. The best exercise is the one you'll actually do consistently.

## Workplace Wellness and Pain Management

The modern workplace presents numerous challenges for people with chronic pain. Long hours at computers, high stress levels, and sedentary work can all contribute to pain and dysfunction. However, strategic workplace modifications can transform your work environment from a source of pain into a tool for healing.

## Ergonomic Fundamentals

Your workstation setup directly affects your pain levels, particularly for neck, back, and wrist pain. Proper monitor height, chair adjustment, and keyboard positioning can prevent many work-related pain problems.

The monitor should be positioned so that the top of the screen is at or slightly below eye level. This positioning prevents neck strain from looking up or down at the screen. The monitor should also be about arm's length away to prevent eye strain.

Chair height should allow your feet to rest flat on the floor with your knees at about 90 degrees. The chair should provide adequate lumbar support to maintain the natural curve of your lower back. Armrests should support your arms without forcing your shoulders upward.

## Micro-Breaks and Movement

Regular movement throughout the workday is essential for preventing pain and stiffness. The human body isn't designed for prolonged sitting, and even people without chronic pain develop problems from excessive sitting.

The 20-20-20 rule provides a simple framework: every 20 minutes, look at something 20 feet away for 20 seconds. This practice helps prevent eye strain and provides a natural break from focused work.

Movement breaks should include standing, stretching, and walking when possible. Even simple movements like shoulder rolls, neck stretches, and ankle circles can help prevent stiffness and improve circulation.

**Case Example: David's Workplace Modifications**

David, a 45-year-old accountant with chronic neck pain, found that his symptoms worsened dramatically during busy work periods. The combination of stress, poor posture, and long hours at his computer created a perfect storm for pain flares.

David's occupational therapist evaluated his workspace and identified several problems. His monitor was too low, forcing him to look down and creating neck strain. His chair lacked proper lumbar support, and his keyboard was positioned in a way that caused wrist strain.

Simple modifications made a significant difference. David raised his monitor to proper height using a monitor stand, adjusted his chair to provide better support, and repositioned his keyboard and mouse to maintain neutral wrist positions.

David also implemented a structured break schedule that included standing and moving every 30 minutes. He set computer reminders to ensure he took these breaks even during busy periods. The breaks helped prevent the muscle tension that contributed to his pain.

The workplace modifications were supplemented with stress management techniques. David learned to recognize early signs of tension and would use brief relaxation exercises at his desk. These techniques helped prevent stress-related muscle tension.

After implementing these changes, David's work-related pain decreased by 60%. He was able to work longer hours when necessary without experiencing the severe pain flares that had previously been inevitable during busy periods.

## Stress Management at Work

Workplace stress can significantly worsen chronic pain through multiple mechanisms. Stress hormones increase inflammation and pain sensitivity, while muscle tension from stress can create additional pain. Managing workplace stress is therefore essential for pain management.

Simple breathing exercises can be done at your desk and provide immediate stress relief. Deep breathing activates the relaxation response and can help prevent stress-related muscle tension.

Time management skills can reduce the sense of overwhelm that contributes to workplace stress. This might involve prioritizing tasks, setting realistic deadlines, and learning to say no to excessive demands.

## Communication with Supervisors

Many people with chronic pain hesitate to discuss their condition with supervisors, fearing discrimination or job loss. However, open communication can often lead to accommodations that benefit both you and your employer.

Focus on solutions rather than problems when discussing your needs. Instead of emphasizing limitations, propose specific accommodations that would help you perform your job more effectively.

Documentation of your condition and accommodation needs can be helpful if formal requests are necessary. This might involve letters from healthcare providers or information about your specific requirements.

## Evening Wind-Down Routines

How you end your day is just as important as how you start it. Evening routines prepare your body and mind for restorative sleep while helping you process the day's stresses and pains. A well-designed evening routine can significantly improve sleep quality and reduce next-day pain levels.

## The Pain-Sleep Connection

Poor sleep increases pain sensitivity and interferes with the body's natural healing processes. Conversely, pain can disrupt sleep quality, creating a vicious cycle that perpetuates both problems. Breaking this cycle requires addressing both sleep quality and pain management.

Your body's natural circadian rhythm influences both sleep and pain sensitivity. Disrupted sleep-wake cycles can worsen pain, while consistent sleep schedules can help regulate pain levels.

## Creating Your Evening Routine

Start your wind-down routine at least one hour before bedtime. This gives your body time to transition from the activity of the day to the restfulness needed for sleep. The routine should be relaxing and signal to your body that it's time to prepare for sleep.

Heat therapy can be particularly beneficial in the evening. A warm bath or shower can help relax tight muscles and reduce pain. The drop in body temperature after leaving the warm water also helps trigger sleepiness.

Gentle stretching or yoga can help release tension accumulated during the day. Focus on areas that tend to hold stress, such as the neck, shoulders, and back. The movement should be gentle and relaxing rather than energizing.

## Case Example: Lisa's Evening Transformation

Lisa, a 38-year-old teacher with fibromyalgia, struggled with severe sleep problems that worsened her pain and fatigue. She would often lie awake for hours, her mind racing with thoughts about work and worries about her health.

Lisa's sleep specialist recommended developing a structured evening routine that would help her transition from the day's activities to restful sleep. The routine needed to address both her physical symptoms and the anxiety that was interfering with sleep.

Lisa began her routine with a warm bath containing Epsom salts. The heat helped relax her muscles, while the magnesium in the salts provided additional relaxation benefits. She used this time for gentle stretching and deep breathing exercises.

The routine also included preparing for the next day to reduce bedtime anxiety. Lisa would lay out her clothes, prepare her lunch, and review her schedule. This preparation helped calm her mind and reduce the worried thoughts that often kept her awake.

Lisa created a sleep-conducive environment by keeping her bedroom cool, dark, and quiet. She invested in blackout curtains and a white noise machine to block out disruptive sounds. These environmental modifications significantly improved her sleep quality.

After implementing her evening routine, Lisa's sleep quality improved dramatically. She fell asleep more easily, stayed asleep longer, and woke up feeling more rested. The improved sleep had a direct impact on her pain levels and overall quality of life.

**Technology and Sleep**

Electronic devices can significantly interfere with sleep quality through blue light exposure and mental stimulation. The blue light from screens can suppress melatonin production and disrupt circadian rhythms.

Establish a technology cutoff time at least one hour before bed. This allows your brain to begin producing melatonin naturally and reduces the mental stimulation that can interfere with sleep.

If you must use devices in the evening, consider blue light filtering glasses or apps that reduce blue light emission. These tools can help minimize the sleep-disrupting effects of technology.

**Relaxation Techniques**

Progressive muscle relaxation involves systematically tensing and releasing muscle groups throughout the body. This technique helps identify areas of tension while promoting overall relaxation.

Guided imagery can help redirect your mind from daily worries to peaceful, relaxing scenes. Many apps and recordings are available that provide guided imagery specifically designed for sleep.

Breathing exercises can help activate the parasympathetic nervous system and promote relaxation. Simple techniques like the 4-7-8 breath can be particularly effective for promoting sleep.

### Weekend Recovery Strategies

Weekends provide opportunities for recovery and restoration that can significantly impact your pain levels during the following week. However, many people with chronic pain struggle with weekends because changes in routine can disrupt their pain management strategies.

### Active Recovery Principles

Active recovery involves engaging in gentle activities that promote healing without adding stress to your system. This might include walking, swimming, gentle yoga, or other low-impact activities that feel good and support your overall health.

The key is finding the right balance between rest and activity. Complete rest can lead to stiffness and deconditioning, while excessive activity can trigger pain flares. Active recovery helps maintain fitness and function while allowing your body to heal.

### Maintaining Routine While Allowing Flexibility

While weekends should provide a break from work stress, maintaining some routine elements can help prevent pain flares. This might include consistent sleep schedules, regular meals, and continued medication schedules.

However, weekends should also allow for some flexibility and enjoyment. The goal is finding a balance that supports your pain management while allowing you to enjoy life and engage in meaningful activities.

**Case Example: Robert's Weekend Balance**

Robert, a 51-year-old with chronic back pain, found that his pain levels spiked every Monday after weekends of either complete inactivity or excessive activity. He couldn't find the right balance between rest and activity.

Robert's physical therapist helped him develop a weekend plan that included structured activities designed to promote recovery while maintaining his fitness. The plan included gentle exercise, stress management, and enjoyable activities that didn't worsen his pain.

Saturday mornings became Robert's time for gentle exercise, such as swimming or walking. These activities helped maintain his fitness while providing pain relief through movement and endorphin release.

Robert also used weekends for activities that he enjoyed but couldn't do during the week, such as spending time in his garden or working on hobbies. These activities provided mental stimulation and stress relief while incorporating gentle movement.

The weekend plan also included time for relaxation and stress management. Robert would use this time for meditation, reading, or other activities that helped him decompress from the week's stresses.

After implementing his weekend recovery plan, Robert's Monday pain levels decreased significantly. He felt more prepared to face the work week and had more energy for both work and personal activities.

**Travel Tips for Pain Management**

Travel can be particularly challenging for people with chronic pain, disrupting routines and creating new stressors. However, with proper planning and strategies, travel can be enjoyable and manageable even with chronic pain conditions.

## Pre-Travel Planning

Research your destination to understand what accommodations and resources will be available. This might include medical facilities, pharmacies, and equipment rental companies if you need special items.

Pack a comprehensive pain management kit that includes medications, heat/cold packs, comfortable clothing, and any devices you use for pain management. Consider bringing extra supplies in case of delays or emergencies.

Plan your itinerary to include rest periods and avoid overexertion. Build flexibility into your schedule to accommodate bad pain days or unexpected symptoms.

## Managing Pain During Travel

Long periods of sitting during flights or car rides can worsen pain and stiffness. Plan to move regularly during travel, even if it's just simple stretches or walking up and down the aisle.

Compression garments can help reduce swelling and pain during long flights. They're particularly beneficial for people with circulation problems or conditions that cause swelling.

Stay hydrated during travel, as dehydration can worsen pain and stiffness. Avoid excessive alcohol consumption, which can interfere with pain medications and disrupt sleep.

## Case Example: Margaret's Travel Success

Margaret, a 59-year-old with arthritis, had stopped traveling because her pain would flare severely during trips. She missed visiting family and friends and felt isolated by her condition.

Margaret's rheumatologist helped her develop a travel plan that addressed her specific needs. The plan included medication timing, movement strategies, and accommodation requests that would help her manage her arthritis while traveling.

Margaret learned to request aisle seats on flights so she could get up and move regularly. She also brought a small pillow and heating pad to help manage stiffness during long flights.

The travel plan included a detailed packing list that ensured Margaret brought all necessary medications and supplies. She learned to pack medications in carry-on luggage to avoid problems if checked bags were delayed.

Margaret also researched her destinations to identify medical facilities and pharmacies in case she needed care while traveling. This preparation gave her confidence and peace of mind during trips.

After implementing her travel plan, Margaret was able to resume traveling and visiting family and friends. She felt more confident about managing her condition while away from home and was able to enjoy travel again.

**Daily Life Integration**

The key to successful pain management lies in integrating evidence-based strategies into your daily routine in ways that feel natural and sustainable. This isn't about adding burden to your life - it's about making choices that support your health and well-being.

Small changes consistently applied often produce better results than dramatic changes that are difficult to maintain. Focus on building habits that become automatic rather than requiring constant willpower and decision-making.

The goal is creating a lifestyle that supports your pain management goals while allowing you to enjoy life and engage in meaningful activities. This balance is different for everyone and may require experimentation to find what works best for your specific situation.

**Living Well with Pain**

The next chapter will explore advanced strategies and future directions in pain management, helping you stay current with new developments and prepare for long-term success in managing your condition.

**Daily Life Mastery**

Integrating pain management into your daily life transforms it from a medical treatment into a way of living. The most effective pain management strategies are those that become natural parts of your routine rather than additional burdens you must carry.

Success comes from understanding that every aspect of your daily life affects your pain levels and overall well-being. From the moment you wake up until you go to sleep, your choices either support healing or perpetuate suffering. The power to influence your pain experience lies in these daily decisions.

**Daily Integration Strategies:**

- Morning routines that address stiffness and prepare your body for the day ahead

- Workplace modifications that prevent pain while supporting productivity

- Evening wind-down routines that promote restorative sleep and recovery

- Weekend recovery strategies that balance rest and activity for optimal healing

- Travel planning that maintains pain management while allowing for life enjoyment

- Sustainable lifestyle changes that support long-term pain management success

# Chapter 18: Post-Surgical and Acute Pain Without Opioids

Surgery represents one of the most challenging scenarios for non-opioid pain management, yet it's also where the benefits of multimodal approaches shine brightest. The traditional approach of relying heavily on opioids for post-operative pain has created widespread addiction problems while often providing inadequate pain relief. Modern evidence-based approaches show that combining multiple non-opioid treatments can provide superior pain control with fewer side effects and complications.

The key to successful surgical pain management lies in planning that begins before the first incision is made. This proactive approach, known as multimodal analgesia, addresses pain through multiple pathways simultaneously, providing more complete relief than any single approach alone. Research published in NCBI and Surgery journals has documented the superior outcomes achieved through these methods (102, 103, 104).

## Multimodal Pre-operative Planning

The foundation of successful surgical pain management is established before you enter the operating room. Pre-operative planning involves assembling a toolkit of pain management strategies that can be implemented at different stages of your surgical journey. This approach recognizes that surgical pain involves multiple mechanisms that require targeted interventions.

## Understanding Surgical Pain Mechanisms

Surgical pain involves tissue damage, inflammation, and nerve sensitization. Each of these mechanisms responds to different treatments, making combination approaches more effective than single interventions. The goal is to prevent pain signals from developing rather than simply treating them after they occur.

Tissue damage creates direct nociceptive pain through activation of pain receptors. Inflammation amplifies these signals while creating additional pain through chemical mediators. Nerve sensitization can cause pain signals to persist even after tissue healing is complete.

## Pre-operative Optimization

Your overall health status before surgery significantly impacts your pain experience and recovery. Optimizing factors like nutrition, sleep, and stress levels can improve surgical outcomes and reduce post-operative pain.

Nutritional status affects wound healing and immune function. Protein is particularly important for tissue repair, while vitamins C and D support immune function and bone healing. Addressing nutritional deficiencies before surgery can improve outcomes.

Sleep quality before surgery influences pain sensitivity and recovery. Poor sleep increases pain sensitivity and impairs immune function. Improving sleep quality in the weeks before surgery can reduce post-operative pain and complications.

## Case Example: Jennifer's Proactive Approach

Jennifer, a 54-year-old teacher, was scheduled for knee replacement surgery after years of arthritis pain. Her orthopedic surgeon recommended a multimodal approach that began several weeks before surgery to optimize her outcomes.

The pre-operative plan included nutritional optimization with protein supplementation and vitamin D correction. Jennifer worked with a dietitian to ensure adequate nutrition for healing while addressing her vitamin D deficiency that could impair bone healing.

Jennifer also began a pre-operative exercise program designed to strengthen the muscles around her knee and improve her overall fitness. This "prehabilitation" approach helped her enter surgery in better physical condition, which improved her recovery.

Pain management education was a crucial component of Jennifer's preparation. She learned about different pain management techniques and set realistic expectations for her recovery. This education reduced her anxiety and helped her prepare mentally for the surgical experience.

The anesthesiologist met with Jennifer before surgery to discuss her pain management plan. They reviewed her medical history, current medications, and pain management preferences. This consultation allowed them to develop a personalized approach to her care.

Jennifer's proactive approach resulted in better pain control and faster recovery than she had expected. Her preparation paid off in reduced post-operative pain and earlier return to normal activities.

## Medication Planning

Pre-operative medication planning involves selecting drugs that can be started before surgery to prevent pain rather than just treating it afterward. This approach can significantly reduce the amount of opioids needed post-operatively.

Anti-inflammatory medications can be started before surgery to reduce the inflammatory response to tissue damage. These medications work best when present in the system before inflammation begins rather than being added afterward.

Nerve-stabilizing medications like gabapentin can be started before surgery to prevent nerve sensitization. These medications take time to reach effective levels, making pre-operative administration beneficial.

Regional anesthesia planning involves determining which nerve blocks or other regional techniques will be most beneficial for your specific surgery. These techniques can provide prolonged pain relief that extends well into the post-operative period.

## Hospital Protocols and Patient Advocacy

Hospitals are increasingly adopting enhanced recovery after surgery (ERAS) protocols that emphasize multimodal pain management. However, not all facilities have implemented these approaches, and you may need to advocate for evidence-based care.

**What to Request from Your Surgical Team**

Ask about multimodal pain management protocols that minimize opioid use. Many hospitals now have standardized approaches that combine different medications and techniques for optimal pain control.

Regional anesthesia should be considered for most surgical procedures. Nerve blocks, spinal anesthesia, and other regional techniques can provide excellent pain relief with minimal side effects.

Request information about the specific medications and techniques that will be used for your pain management. Understanding your treatment plan helps you prepare and make informed decisions about your care.

**Case Example: Robert's Hospital Advocacy**

Robert, a 61-year-old construction worker, was scheduled for rotator cuff repair surgery. He was concerned about opioid use due to a family history of addiction and wanted to explore alternatives.

Robert researched multimodal pain management approaches and discussed them with his orthopedic surgeon. The surgeon was supportive and referred him to an anesthesiologist who specialized in regional anesthesia techniques.

The anesthesiologist recommended a combination of nerve blocks and non-opioid medications for Robert's surgery. This approach would provide excellent pain relief while minimizing opioid requirements.

Robert also asked about the hospital's ERAS protocols and what services would be available to support his recovery. He learned about physical therapy services, nutrition support, and other resources that could help optimize his outcomes.

The surgical team worked together to implement Robert's multimodal pain management plan. The approach was successful, providing good pain control with minimal opioid use and faster recovery than expected.

### Understanding Hospital Pain Management Policies

Many hospitals have moved away from the "pain as the fifth vital sign" approach that contributed to excessive opioid prescribing. New policies emphasize functional goals and multimodal approaches to pain management.

Ask about your hospital's pain management policies and what alternatives are available if standard protocols don't work for you. Understanding these policies helps you advocate for appropriate care.

Some hospitals have acute pain services that specialize in post-operative pain management. These services can provide expertise in complex pain management situations and alternative approaches.

### Home Recovery Without Opioids

The transition from hospital to home represents a critical period in surgical recovery. Having a well-planned approach to home pain management can prevent complications and reduce the need for opioid medications.

### Creating Your Home Pain Management Kit

Assemble supplies before your surgery so they're available when you need them. This should include ice packs, heating pads, comfortable clothing, and any recommended devices or equipment.

Non-prescription medications like acetaminophen and ibuprofen can provide significant pain relief when used appropriately. Understanding proper dosing and timing helps maximize their effectiveness.

Topical pain medications can provide localized relief without systemic side effects. These medications work best when applied regularly rather than just when pain is severe.

**Case Example: Susan's Home Recovery Success**

Susan, a 47-year-old nurse, had gallbladder surgery and wanted to minimize opioid use during her recovery. She developed a detailed home recovery plan that focused on non-opioid pain management strategies.

Susan's kit included multiple ice packs for rotation, a heating pad for muscle tension, and comfortable clothing that wouldn't irritate her surgical sites. She also had a variety of pillows for positioning and support.

The medication plan included scheduled acetaminophen and ibuprofen, taken at regular intervals rather than waiting for pain to become severe. This approach provided consistent pain relief throughout her recovery.

Susan also prepared easy-to-prepare meals and arranged for help with household tasks. This preparation allowed her to focus on recovery rather than daily responsibilities that might worsen her pain.

Her home recovery plan was successful, providing good pain control without opioids. Susan felt more in control of her recovery and experienced fewer side effects than she had expected.

**Activity and Movement Guidelines**

Early mobilization is crucial for preventing complications and reducing pain. However, the type and intensity of activity must be appropriate for your specific surgery and recovery stage.

Walking is generally safe and beneficial after most surgeries. Start with short distances and gradually increase as tolerated. Walking helps prevent complications like blood clots and promotes healing.

Breathing exercises are particularly important after chest or abdominal surgery. These exercises help prevent pneumonia and other respiratory complications while promoting healing.

Position changes help prevent stiffness and pressure sores. Change positions regularly, even if movement is uncomfortable initially. This prevents problems that could worsen pain later.

### Physical Therapy Timeline and Implementation

Physical therapy plays a crucial role in surgical recovery, but timing and intensity must be carefully managed. Research published in PLOS has documented the importance of early, appropriate physical therapy in preventing chronic pain after surgery (105).

### Early Post-operative Phase

The first 48-72 hours after surgery focus on preventing complications and beginning gentle movement. This might include breathing exercises, ankle pumps, and position changes rather than formal exercise.

Pain management during early physical therapy is crucial for success. Timing therapy sessions with pain medication can improve participation and outcomes.

### Progressive Mobilization

As healing progresses, physical therapy becomes more active and focused on restoring function. The progression must be gradual to avoid complications while promoting optimal recovery.

Range of motion exercises help prevent stiffness and maintain joint flexibility. These exercises should be performed regularly, even if they cause mild discomfort initially.

Strengthening exercises are gradually added as healing allows. The focus is on rebuilding strength lost during the recovery period while protecting healing tissues.

## Case Example: Michael's Physical Therapy Success

Michael, a 52-year-old accountant, had spinal fusion surgery and was concerned about his ability to return to work. His surgeon recommended an aggressive physical therapy program to optimize his recovery.

Physical therapy began in the hospital with basic mobility exercises and proper body mechanics training. The focus was on moving safely while protecting his surgical site.

As Michael progressed, therapy became more intensive, focusing on core strengthening and functional activities. The program was individualized based on his specific needs and recovery progress.

Michael's commitment to physical therapy paid off in faster recovery and better functional outcomes. He was able to return to work sooner than expected with good pain control.

## Functional Goals and Milestones

Physical therapy should focus on functional goals rather than just pain reduction. This approach helps ensure that you regain the ability to perform activities that are important to you.

Milestones help track progress and provide motivation during recovery. These might include walking specific distances, climbing stairs, or performing work-related activities.

Communication with your physical therapist is crucial for success. Report any problems or concerns promptly so adjustments can be made to your treatment plan.

## Preventing Chronic Pain After Surgery

The transition from acute post-operative pain to chronic pain represents a critical period that requires careful management. Early interventions can prevent the development of chronic pain conditions that can persist long after surgical healing is complete.

## Understanding the Risk Factors

Certain factors increase the risk of developing chronic pain after surgery. These include pre-existing pain conditions, anxiety, depression, and certain types of surgeries that involve significant nerve manipulation.

The intensity and duration of acute post-operative pain can influence the development of chronic pain. Aggressive pain management during the acute phase may help prevent chronicity.

## Early Intervention Strategies

Multimodal pain management during the acute phase can help prevent central sensitization that leads to chronic pain. This approach addresses pain through multiple mechanisms simultaneously.

Psychological support during recovery can help address fear, anxiety, and depression that contribute to chronic pain development. These factors can be addressed through counseling or stress management techniques.

## Case Example: Lisa's Prevention Success

Lisa, a 43-year-old teacher, had breast cancer surgery and was at high risk for developing chronic pain due to the extensive nature of her procedure. Her surgical team implemented aggressive prevention strategies.

The prevention plan included optimal pain management during the acute phase, early mobilization, and psychological support. Lisa also received education about chronic pain prevention and warning signs to watch for.

Physical therapy began early and focused on preventing the movement restrictions that could contribute to chronic pain. The program included gentle stretching, strengthening, and scar tissue management.

Lisa's prevention strategies were successful, and she avoided the chronic pain complications that affect many patients after similar surgeries. Her proactive approach contributed to better long-term outcomes.

## Long-term Monitoring

Regular follow-up is important for detecting early signs of chronic pain development. This monitoring allows for early intervention if problems develop.

Pain that persists beyond the expected healing time should be evaluated promptly. Early treatment of persistent pain can prevent it from becoming chronic.

## Opioid Alternatives in Emergency Situations

Even with the best planning, some situations may require additional pain management interventions. Understanding alternatives to opioids for breakthrough pain can help you avoid unnecessary opioid exposure.

## Breakthrough Pain Management

Breakthrough pain can occur even with good baseline pain management. Having a plan for managing these episodes helps prevent panic and ensures appropriate treatment.

Additional non-opioid medications can often manage breakthrough pain effectively. This might include additional anti-inflammatory drugs or topical medications.

## When Opioids Might Be Necessary

While the goal is to avoid opioids, there are situations where they may be medically necessary. Understanding these situations helps you make informed decisions about your care.

If opioids are necessary, they should be used for the shortest duration possible and with a clear plan for discontinuation. This approach minimizes risks while providing necessary pain relief.

## Surgical Recovery Mastery

The next chapter will explore special populations and the unique considerations required for effective pain management in children, elderly patients, pregnant women, athletes, and people with multiple chronic conditions.

## Recovery Without Dependency

Post-surgical pain management without opioids is not only possible but often superior to traditional approaches. The key lies in comprehensive planning that begins before surgery and continues through recovery. By understanding the mechanisms of surgical pain and implementing evidence-based interventions, you can achieve excellent pain control while avoiding the risks associated with opioid medications.

Success requires active participation in your care, from pre-operative optimization through home recovery. The multimodal approach addresses pain through multiple pathways, providing more complete relief than any single intervention. This strategy, combined with appropriate physical therapy and chronic pain prevention measures, can lead to faster recovery and better long-term outcomes.

**Post-Surgical Pain Management Essentials:**

- Pre-operative planning and optimization set the foundation for successful recovery

- Hospital protocols should include multimodal approaches that minimize opioid requirements

- Home recovery toolkits provide effective alternatives to opioid medications

- Physical therapy timing and progression are crucial for optimal functional recovery

- Early intervention strategies can prevent the development of chronic post-surgical pain

- Breakthrough pain can usually be managed with non-opioid alternatives when properly planned

# Chapter 19: Special Populations and Considerations

Pain management is not a one-size-fits-all approach. Different populations require modified strategies that account for unique physiological, psychological, and social factors. Children process pain differently than adults, elderly patients have different risk factors and medication sensitivities, and pregnant women require treatments that are safe for both mother and baby. Understanding these differences is essential for safe, effective pain management across all populations.

This chapter addresses the specific considerations needed for pediatric patients, elderly individuals, pregnant women, athletes, and people managing multiple chronic conditions. Each population presents unique challenges and opportunities that require tailored approaches to achieve optimal outcomes.

## Pediatric Pain Management

Children's pain has been historically undertreated due to misconceptions about how children experience and express pain. We now understand that children feel pain as intensely as adults, and undertreated pain can have lasting effects on their development and future pain experiences.

## Understanding Pediatric Pain Differences

Children's nervous systems are still developing, which affects how they process and respond to pain. Very young children may not have the language skills to describe their pain, requiring healthcare providers and parents to rely on behavioral indicators.

Pain expression varies significantly with age. Infants may show pain through crying, changes in sleep patterns, or decreased feeding. Toddlers might become irritable or regress in their development. School-age children can often describe their pain but may minimize it to avoid medical procedures.

## Safe Pain Management Approaches

Non-pharmacological approaches are often the first line of treatment for pediatric pain. These include comfort measures, distraction techniques, and age-appropriate coping strategies that help children manage their pain experience.

Distraction techniques can be remarkably effective for children. This might include toys, games, music, or videos that capture the child's attention and reduce their focus on pain.

Comfort measures like positioning, swaddling for infants, or the presence of parents can significantly reduce pain perception in children. These interventions work by providing security and reducing anxiety.

## Case Example: Emma's Pediatric Pain Journey

Emma, a 7-year-old girl, required surgery for a broken arm. Her parents were concerned about pain management and wanted to minimize medication use while ensuring their daughter's comfort.

The pediatric team developed a comprehensive pain management plan that included both pharmacological and non-pharmacological approaches. The plan was explained to Emma in age-appropriate language to reduce her anxiety.

Pre-operative preparation included a hospital tour and child life specialist interaction. Emma was able to see the operating room and meet the surgical team, which reduced her fear and anxiety about the procedure.

Pain management included child-friendly techniques like "magic" numbing cream for IV insertion and the use of nitrous oxide for procedures. These approaches made medical care less frightening for Emma.

The post-operative plan included scheduled pain medication, ice therapy, and distraction activities. Emma's parents were taught to recognize signs of pain and how to implement comfort measures.

Emma's recovery was successful, with good pain control and minimal distress. The family-centered approach helped both Emma and her parents feel more in control of the situation.

## Family-Centered Care

Parents play a crucial role in pediatric pain management. They know their child best and can identify subtle changes that might indicate pain or distress.

Education for parents about pain assessment and management helps them become effective advocates for their children. This includes understanding when to seek help and how to implement comfort measures.

Involving siblings and other family members in age-appropriate ways can help reduce the child's stress and improve their coping with pain.

## Elderly Pain Management

Aging brings unique challenges to pain management, including multiple chronic conditions, medication interactions, and changes in drug metabolism. UCLA Health has published research on age-specific pain management strategies that address these complex needs (106).

## Age-Related Changes in Pain Processing

Older adults may experience changes in pain perception due to aging nervous systems. Some may have decreased pain sensitivity, while others may experience increased sensitivity due to conditions like neuropathy.

Multiple chronic conditions are common in elderly patients, making pain management more complex. Arthritis, diabetes, heart disease, and other conditions can all contribute to pain while affecting treatment options.

## Medication Considerations

Older adults metabolize medications differently than younger people, often requiring lower doses or different medications to achieve the same effects. Kidney and liver function decline with age, affecting how drugs are processed.

Polypharmacy - taking multiple medications - is common in elderly patients and increases the risk of drug interactions. Pain medications must be carefully selected to avoid interactions with other prescribed drugs.

## Case Example: Robert's Geriatric Pain Management

Robert, a 78-year-old retired teacher, developed multiple pain conditions including arthritis, neuropathy, and chronic back pain. His primary care physician struggled to manage his complex pain while avoiding medication interactions.

Robert's medication list included treatments for diabetes, heart disease, and high blood pressure. Adding pain medications required careful consideration of potential interactions and side effects.

The geriatric pain management approach focused on non-pharmacological interventions as the foundation of care. This included physical therapy, occupational therapy, and lifestyle modifications that addressed multiple conditions simultaneously.

When medications were necessary, they were started at low doses and increased gradually. Robert's response was monitored closely, and adjustments were made based on his individual response.

The team approach included Robert's family members, who helped monitor his response to treatments and provided support for lifestyle modifications. This support was crucial for maintaining his independence.

Robert's complex pain conditions were successfully managed through the multimodal approach. His quality of life improved, and he was able to maintain his independence at home.

### Fall Prevention and Safety

Pain medications can increase fall risk in elderly patients, making safety a primary concern. Balance, cognitive function, and reaction times can all be affected by pain medications.

Environmental modifications can help reduce fall risk while supporting pain management. This might include grab bars, improved lighting, and removal of trip hazards.

### Cognitive Considerations

Dementia and other cognitive impairments affect pain assessment and management in elderly patients. These patients may not be able to communicate their pain effectively or understand treatment instructions.

Behavioral indicators become more important for pain assessment in patients with cognitive impairment. Changes in activity level, agitation, or sleep patterns may indicate pain.

### Pregnancy and Pain Management

Pregnancy creates unique challenges for pain management, as treatments must be safe for both mother and developing baby. The Cleveland Clinic has published guidance on safe pain management approaches during pregnancy (107).

### Physiological Changes During Pregnancy

Pregnancy causes significant changes in how the body processes medications. Blood volume increases, kidney function changes, and liver metabolism is altered, all affecting drug levels and effectiveness.

Hormonal changes during pregnancy can affect pain sensitivity and muscle function. The hormone relaxin, which helps prepare the body for childbirth, can cause joint instability and pain.

### Safe Treatment Options

Non-pharmacological approaches are preferred during pregnancy when possible. These include physical therapy, massage, heat therapy, and relaxation techniques that are safe for both mother and baby.

Acetaminophen is generally considered safe during pregnancy and can be effective for many types of pain. However, even this medication should be used at the lowest effective dose.

## Case Example: Sarah's Pregnancy Pain Management

Sarah, a 32-year-old marketing manager, developed severe back pain during her second trimester of pregnancy. The pain was affecting her ability to work and sleep, but she was concerned about medication effects on her baby.

Sarah's obstetrician referred her to a physical therapist who specialized in pregnancy-related pain. The therapist developed a program that was safe for her pregnancy stage and addressed her specific pain issues.

The treatment plan included prenatal yoga, specific exercises for back pain, and postural education. Sarah also learned proper body mechanics for daily activities that could reduce her pain.

A pregnancy support belt helped reduce the load on Sarah's back while providing stability. This simple intervention provided significant relief without any risk to the baby.

Sarah also received education about pain management during labor and delivery. This preparation helped her make informed decisions about her birth plan and pain management options.

The pregnancy pain management approach was successful, allowing Sarah to remain active throughout her pregnancy. She felt confident in her pain management decisions and had a positive birth experience.

## Labor and Delivery Considerations

Pain management during labor and delivery requires balancing maternal comfort with baby safety. Many effective options are available that meet both criteria.

Epidural anesthesia is commonly used and generally safe when administered by skilled providers. This technique can provide excellent pain relief while allowing the mother to remain alert and participate in the birth.

Non-pharmacological approaches like breathing techniques, positioning, and water therapy can be effective for labor pain. These methods have no medication risks and can be combined with other approaches.

### Postpartum Pain Management

Pain after childbirth requires special consideration, especially for breastfeeding mothers. Medications can pass into breast milk and affect the baby.

Many pain medications are compatible with breastfeeding, but dosing and timing may need adjustment. Healthcare providers can help mothers make informed decisions about pain management while breastfeeding.

### Athletes and Active Individuals

Athletes present unique challenges for pain management due to their high activity levels, performance demands, and risk of injury. Treatment approaches must address pain while maintaining or restoring athletic performance.

### Understanding Athletic Pain

Athletes may experience both acute injuries and chronic overuse conditions. The demands of training and competition can make rest-based treatments challenging to implement.

Pain tolerance may be different in athletes, who are often trained to push through discomfort. This can lead to underreporting of pain or inappropriate activity levels during recovery.

### Performance-Focused Treatment Approaches

Athletic pain management must consider the athlete's sport, position, and competition schedule. Treatments should be timed to minimize impact on performance while providing adequate pain relief.

Functional movement assessment helps identify biomechanical issues that contribute to pain. Correcting these issues can provide pain relief while improving performance.

**Case Example: Jake's Sports Medicine Approach**

Jake, a 24-year-old college baseball pitcher, developed shoulder pain that was affecting his performance. He was concerned about missing games and wanted treatment that would allow him to continue playing.

The sports medicine team performed a comprehensive evaluation that included movement analysis, strength testing, and injury assessment. They identified specific biomechanical issues that were contributing to Jake's pain.

The treatment plan included targeted physical therapy to address the biomechanical issues, along with pain management techniques that didn't interfere with his performance. The approach was designed to provide relief while improving his pitching mechanics.

Jake also received education about injury prevention and proper warm-up techniques. This knowledge helped him reduce his risk of future injuries while maintaining his performance level.

The sports medicine approach was successful, allowing Jake to continue playing while addressing his pain. His performance actually improved as his biomechanical issues were corrected.

**Return-to-Play Decisions**

Determining when an athlete can safely return to activity requires careful assessment of healing, function, and risk factors. This decision involves balancing athletic goals with long-term health.

Graduated return-to-play protocols help ensure that athletes are ready for the demands of their sport. These protocols progressively increase activity levels while monitoring for symptom recurrence.

## Doping and Supplement Considerations

Athletes must be careful about pain medications and supplements that might contain banned substances. Many common pain medications are prohibited in competitive sports.

Working with sports medicine professionals who understand anti-doping regulations helps ensure that pain management approaches are both effective and compliant with athletic regulations.

## Managing Multiple Chronic Conditions

People with multiple chronic conditions face complex pain management challenges. Treatments must address various conditions simultaneously while avoiding harmful interactions.

## Condition Interactions

Multiple conditions can interact in ways that complicate pain management. Diabetes can cause neuropathy, arthritis can limit mobility, and heart disease can restrict medication options.

Understanding these interactions helps healthcare providers develop treatment plans that address all conditions while minimizing conflicts between treatments.

## Coordinated Care Approaches

Managing multiple conditions requires coordination between various healthcare providers. This coordination helps ensure that treatments complement rather than interfere with each other.

A primary care physician often serves as the coordinator for complex cases, ensuring that all providers are aware of the patient's complete medical picture.

## Case Example: Maria's Complex Condition Management

Maria, a 68-year-old retired nurse, had diabetes, arthritis, heart disease, and chronic pain from a previous back injury. Her multiple conditions made pain management challenging and required careful coordination.

Maria's primary care physician worked with specialists to develop a coordinated treatment plan. Each provider was aware of her complete medical history and current treatments.

The pain management approach focused on treatments that could address multiple conditions simultaneously. Physical therapy helped with both arthritis and back pain, while dietary modifications supported diabetes management and weight loss.

Medication management required careful consideration of interactions and side effects. Maria's heart condition limited some pain medication options, while her diabetes required monitoring of blood sugar levels.

The coordinated approach was successful in managing Maria's complex conditions. Her pain levels decreased, and her overall health improved through the integrated treatment plan.

## Medication Management Complexity

Multiple chronic conditions often require multiple medications, increasing the complexity of pain management. Drug interactions, side effects, and dosing schedules must all be carefully managed.

Medication reconciliation helps ensure that all providers are aware of current medications and can identify potential problems before they occur.

## Quality of Life Considerations

Multiple chronic conditions can significantly impact quality of life beyond just pain levels. Treatment approaches should address functional limitations, emotional well-being, and social participation.

Goal setting becomes more complex with multiple conditions, requiring prioritization of outcomes and realistic expectations about improvement.

## Population-Specific Success Strategies

The next chapter will explore future directions in pain management, including emerging treatments, personalized medicine approaches, and technological innovations that promise to improve outcomes for all populations.

## Tailored Care Excellence

Managing pain across different populations requires understanding that one size does not fit all. Each group - children, elderly patients, pregnant women, athletes, and those with multiple conditions - presents unique challenges and opportunities that demand specialized approaches.

Success in population-specific pain management comes from recognizing these differences and adapting treatment strategies accordingly. This might mean using different assessment tools, modifying medication dosages, or emphasizing particular non-pharmacological approaches that work best for specific populations.

## Population-Specific Care Principles:

- Pediatric pain management requires age-appropriate approaches and family involvement
- Elderly patients need careful medication management and fall prevention strategies
- Pregnancy pain management prioritizes safety for both mother and baby
- Athletic pain management must balance performance goals with long-term health
- Multiple chronic conditions require coordinated care and careful medication management

- Each population benefits from tailored approaches that address their unique needs and circumstances

# Chapter 20: The Future of Natural Pain Relief

The field of pain management stands at the threshold of remarkable advances that promise to transform how we understand, assess, and treat pain. From precision medicine approaches that tailor treatments to individual genetic profiles to artificial intelligence systems that can predict and prevent pain flares, the future holds unprecedented possibilities for people suffering from chronic pain conditions.

These innovations represent more than incremental improvements - they signal a fundamental shift toward personalized, targeted, and technology-enhanced pain management. The convergence of biological discovery, technological innovation, and data science is creating opportunities that were unimaginable just a decade ago.

## Pipeline Innovations in Pain Medication

The pharmaceutical pipeline for pain management is experiencing a renaissance of innovation, moving beyond traditional opioid-based approaches to target specific pain mechanisms with greater precision and fewer side effects. Research published in Labiotech has highlighted numerous promising compounds in development (108, 109).

## LTG Compounds and Sodium Channel Modulators

The success of suzetrigine (Journavx) has validated the approach of targeting specific sodium channels involved in pain signaling. This breakthrough has opened the door to an entire class of sodium channel modulators that could provide effective pain relief without opioid-related risks.

LTG-001, developed by Latigo Biotherapeutics, represents the next generation of Nav1.8 channel inhibitors. This compound has received FDA Fast Track designation for acute pain treatment, suggesting that regulatory agencies recognize the potential of this approach.

The advantage of sodium channel modulators lies in their specificity. Unlike opioids, which affect multiple body systems, these compounds target the specific pathways involved in pain signaling. This precision reduces side effects while maintaining effectiveness.

## CGRP-Based Innovations

The success of CGRP inhibitors for migraine prevention has sparked development of related compounds for other pain conditions. Researchers are exploring whether CGRP pathways play roles in arthritis, neuropathic pain, and other chronic conditions.

Oral CGRP receptor antagonists are being developed for various pain conditions beyond migraines. These compounds could provide targeted pain relief for conditions that don't respond well to traditional treatments.

## Case Example: Patricia's Clinical Trial Experience

Patricia, a 58-year-old with treatment-resistant neuropathic pain, enrolled in a clinical trial for a novel sodium channel modulator. Traditional treatments had provided minimal relief, and she was interested in exploring new options.

The clinical trial provided Patricia with access to cutting-edge treatment while contributing to medical knowledge. The compound she received was specifically designed to target the type of nerve pain she experienced.

Patricia's experience in the trial was positive, with significant pain reduction and minimal side effects. The targeted approach provided relief that traditional medications hadn't achieved.

The clinical trial also provided Patricia with enhanced medical monitoring and support. This level of care helped optimize her treatment while ensuring her safety throughout the study.

Patricia's participation in the trial not only helped her own pain management but also contributed to the development of treatments that could help thousands of others with similar conditions.

### Regenerative Medicine Approaches

Stem cell therapy and platelet-rich plasma (PRP) treatments represent potentially revolutionary approaches to pain management. These treatments aim to heal damaged tissues rather than just managing symptoms.

However, the field of regenerative medicine is still developing, and many claims about these treatments exceed current scientific evidence. It's important to distinguish between legitimate research and unproven commercial applications.

Current research focuses on understanding which conditions might benefit from regenerative approaches and how to optimize these treatments for maximum effectiveness and safety.

### Personalized Pain Medicine

The future of pain management lies in personalized approaches that consider individual genetic, biological, and psychological factors. This precision medicine approach promises to move beyond trial-and-error treatment selection to evidence-based, individualized care.

### Genetic Testing and Treatment Selection

Genetic variations affect how individuals respond to pain medications, process inflammation, and experience pain sensitivity. Understanding these genetic factors could revolutionize treatment selection.

Pharmacogenetic testing can identify how individuals metabolize specific medications, allowing for more precise dosing and drug selection. This approach could reduce adverse reactions while improving treatment effectiveness.

Pain sensitivity genes are being identified that could help predict which treatments are most likely to be effective for individual patients. This information could guide treatment selection from the beginning rather than through trial and error.

## Biomarker Development

Researchers are developing biological markers that could predict treatment response and monitor progress objectively. These biomarkers could transform pain management from a subjective experience to a measurable medical condition.

Inflammatory markers already help guide treatment for some conditions, and new biomarkers are being developed for various pain conditions. These tools could help optimize treatment timing and selection.

## Case Example: David's Personalized Approach

David, a 52-year-old with complex pain conditions, participated in a personalized pain management program that used genetic testing and biomarker analysis to guide his treatment.

The genetic testing revealed that David metabolized certain pain medications differently than average, explaining why some treatments hadn't worked well for him. This information guided selection of alternative medications.

Biomarker analysis showed that David had elevated inflammatory markers that suggested he would respond well to anti-inflammatory treatments. This information helped prioritize treatments that targeted his specific biological profile.

The personalized approach resulted in better pain control with fewer side effects than David's previous treatments. The targeted selection of therapies based on his individual characteristics improved his outcomes significantly.

David's experience demonstrates the potential of personalized medicine to transform pain management from a one-size-fits-all approach to individualized care.

## Artificial Intelligence in Treatment Selection

Machine learning algorithms are being developed that can analyze complex patterns in patient data to predict treatment responses.

These systems could help healthcare providers make more informed treatment decisions.

AI systems can consider far more variables than human providers, potentially identifying treatment patterns that aren't obvious through traditional clinical assessment.

## Digital Therapeutics and Technology Integration

Technology is transforming pain management through digital therapeutics, smartphone applications, and wearable devices that provide continuous monitoring and intervention capabilities.

## Prescription Digital Therapeutics

Digital therapeutics are evidence-based software programs that can be prescribed like medications. These programs provide structured interventions for pain management, often incorporating cognitive behavioral therapy principles.

The FDA has begun approving digital therapeutics for various conditions, establishing a regulatory framework for these innovative treatments. This approval process ensures that digital therapeutics meet safety and effectiveness standards.

## Smartphone Applications and Monitoring

Smartphone apps are becoming increasingly sophisticated in their ability to track pain patterns, predict flares, and provide real-time interventions. These tools could democratize access to pain management support.

Machine learning algorithms can analyze data from smartphone sensors to identify patterns that predict pain flares. This capability could allow for preventive interventions before pain becomes severe.

## Wearable Technology

Wearable devices are being developed that can continuously monitor physiological parameters related to pain, such as heart rate variability, sleep quality, and activity levels.

These devices could provide objective measures of pain-related dysfunction and treatment response, moving beyond subjective pain ratings to measurable outcomes.

## Case Example: Lisa's Digital Health Journey

Lisa, a 44-year-old with fibromyalgia, used a comprehensive digital health platform that combined smartphone apps, wearable devices, and digital therapeutics to manage her condition.

The platform tracked her sleep, activity, stress levels, and pain patterns to identify triggers and effective interventions. This comprehensive monitoring provided insights that weren't available through traditional clinical assessment.

The digital therapeutic component provided Lisa with access to cognitive behavioral therapy techniques, relaxation training, and educational content tailored to her specific needs and progress.

The wearable device monitored her sleep quality and activity levels, providing objective data about her condition that complemented her subjective pain reports.

Lisa's digital health approach improved her pain management outcomes while providing her with more control over her condition. The technology-enhanced approach supplemented traditional medical care effectively.

## Virtual Reality and Augmented Reality

VR and AR technologies are being developed for pain management applications beyond simple distraction. These tools could provide immersive therapeutic experiences that address multiple aspects of pain.

VR-based physical therapy programs could provide engaging, effective treatment that's more accessible than traditional therapy settings. These programs could be particularly valuable for people with mobility limitations.

## Artificial Intelligence and Machine Learning

AI and machine learning are poised to revolutionize pain management through improved diagnosis, treatment selection, and outcome prediction. These technologies can analyze vast amounts of data to identify patterns that humans might miss.

### Diagnostic Applications

AI systems are being developed that can analyze medical images, patient histories, and other data to improve diagnostic accuracy for pain conditions. These systems could help identify conditions that are currently difficult to diagnose.

Machine learning algorithms can identify patterns in electronic health records that predict which patients are at risk for developing chronic pain, allowing for preventive interventions.

### Treatment Optimization

AI systems can analyze patient responses to different treatments to identify optimal approaches for individual patients. These systems could reduce the trial-and-error approach that currently characterizes much of pain management.

Predictive models could identify which patients are likely to respond to specific treatments, allowing for more targeted therapy selection from the beginning.

### Case Example: Robert's AI-Assisted Care

Robert, a 59-year-old with complex chronic pain, received care at a medical center that used AI-assisted treatment selection. The system analyzed his medical history, genetic profile, and treatment responses to guide care decisions.

The AI system identified patterns in Robert's case that suggested he would respond well to a specific combination of treatments that his providers might not have considered otherwise.

The system also predicted potential side effects and drug interactions, helping Robert's healthcare team avoid problems before they occurred.

Robert's AI-assisted care resulted in better pain control with fewer side effects than his previous treatments. The technology-enhanced approach improved his outcomes significantly.

## Continuous Learning Systems

AI systems can continuously learn from new data, improving their accuracy and effectiveness over time. This capability could lead to constantly improving pain management approaches.

These systems could identify new treatment patterns and effectiveness indicators that weren't previously recognized, advancing the field of pain management.

## Regenerative Medicine Reality Check

While regenerative medicine holds promise for pain management, it's important to distinguish between legitimate research and unproven commercial applications. The field is still developing, and many claims exceed current scientific evidence.

## Stem Cell Therapy

Legitimate stem cell research is exploring how these cells might help repair damaged tissues that cause pain. However, many commercial stem cell clinics offer treatments that haven't been proven safe or effective.

The FDA regulates stem cell treatments, and patients should be wary of clinics offering unproven therapies. Legitimate research is conducted through clinical trials with proper oversight.

## Platelet-Rich Plasma (PRP)

PRP therapy involves injecting concentrated platelets from the patient's own blood into painful areas. Some research suggests benefits for certain conditions, but the evidence is still limited.

The quality of PRP preparation and injection techniques can vary significantly, affecting treatment outcomes. Standardization of these procedures is needed for consistent results.

### Case Example: Michael's Regenerative Medicine Experience

Michael, a 48-year-old athlete with chronic tendon pain, considered regenerative medicine treatments after traditional therapies provided limited relief. He researched his options carefully before making decisions.

Michael chose to participate in a legitimate clinical trial for PRP therapy rather than seeking commercial treatment. The trial provided access to cutting-edge treatment with proper medical oversight.

The clinical trial results were mixed, with some patients experiencing significant improvement while others saw minimal benefit. Michael experienced moderate improvement that allowed him to return to modified athletic activities.

Michael's experience highlights the importance of participating in legitimate research rather than seeking unproven commercial treatments. The clinical trial provided him with access to innovative therapy while contributing to medical knowledge.

### Future Directions

Regenerative medicine research continues to advance, with new approaches being developed and tested. Future treatments may be more effective and predictable than current options.

The key to success in regenerative medicine will be understanding which conditions are most likely to benefit and how to optimize these treatments for maximum effectiveness.

### Staying Informed About Advances

The rapid pace of innovation in pain management makes it important to stay informed about new developments. However, it's equally important to distinguish between legitimate advances and unproven claims.

## Reliable Information Sources

Professional medical organizations provide evidence-based information about new treatments and research developments. These sources can help you stay informed about legitimate advances.

Peer-reviewed medical journals publish research findings that have been evaluated by experts in the field. These sources provide the most reliable information about new treatments.

## Evaluating New Treatments

New treatments should be evaluated based on scientific evidence rather than marketing claims. Look for research published in reputable journals and approved by regulatory agencies.

Be wary of treatments that promise miraculous results or claim to cure all types of pain. Legitimate treatments typically have specific indications and limitations.

## Participating in Research

Clinical trials provide access to cutting-edge treatments while contributing to medical knowledge. Participation in legitimate research can benefit both individual patients and the broader pain management community.

Research participation should be voluntary and well-informed. Patients should understand the potential benefits and risks before agreeing to participate.

## Innovation and Hope

The future of pain management offers unprecedented hope for people suffering from chronic pain conditions. Advances in medication development, personalized medicine, digital therapeutics, and artificial intelligence promise to transform how we understand and treat pain.

These innovations represent more than technological progress - they signal a fundamental shift toward more effective, personalized, and accessible pain management. The convergence of biological discovery, technological innovation, and data science is creating opportunities that could benefit millions of people worldwide.

The key to realizing these benefits lies in continued research, responsible innovation, and patient participation in the development of new treatments. The future of pain management is bright, but it requires ongoing commitment to scientific rigor and patient-centered care.

### Tomorrow's Pain Relief Today

The future of natural pain relief is being written today through innovative research, technological development, and clinical practice. While many promising treatments are still in development, the trajectory is clear - we're moving toward more effective, personalized, and accessible pain management approaches.

Success in this evolving field requires staying informed about legitimate advances while maintaining healthy skepticism about unproven claims. The most promising developments combine scientific rigor with patient-centered care, offering hope for better outcomes while maintaining safety and effectiveness standards.

### Future Directions in Pain Management:

- Pipeline innovations are developing targeted medications with fewer side effects than traditional approaches

- Personalized medicine promises to match treatments to individual genetic and biological profiles

- Digital therapeutics and AI are creating new possibilities for accessible, continuous care

- Regenerative medicine approaches require careful evaluation to distinguish proven from unproven treatments

- Staying informed about advances requires relying on credible sources and scientific evidence

- The future of pain management depends on continued research, innovation, and patient participation

# Appendix A: Quick Reference Guides

Pain doesn't follow a convenient schedule, striking at 3 AM, during important meetings, or when you're miles from home. This appendix provides the essential tools you need for immediate pain relief, safety monitoring, and proper medication management. Think of these guides as your pain management emergency kit - ready when you need them most.

The information here distills complex medical guidance into actionable steps you can follow even when pain is clouding your judgment. Each guide has been designed for clarity and speed, giving you the confidence to act appropriately during pain crises while knowing when professional help is necessary.

**Emergency Pain Relief Techniques**

**Immediate Assessment and Action**

When severe pain strikes, your first priority is determining if this represents a medical emergency. New, sudden, or severe pain requires different responses than familiar chronic pain flares. Start by assessing the pain's characteristics and your overall condition.

For sudden, severe pain accompanied by difficulty breathing, chest tightness, or loss of consciousness, call emergency services immediately. These symptoms suggest potentially life-threatening conditions that require immediate medical attention.

For severe pain without emergency symptoms, begin with the RICE protocol if appropriate: Rest the affected area, apply Ice for 15-20 minutes, apply gentle Compression if swelling is present, and Elevate the affected limb if possible. This approach works best for acute injuries and some chronic pain flares.

**Breathing Techniques for Immediate Relief**

The 4-7-8 breathing technique provides rapid pain relief by activating your body's relaxation response. Inhale through your nose for 4 counts, hold your breath for 7 counts, then exhale through your mouth for 8 counts. Repeat this cycle 3-4 times, then return to normal breathing.

Box breathing offers another powerful technique: Inhale for 4 counts, hold for 4 counts, exhale for 4 counts, hold empty for 4 counts. This pattern helps regulate your nervous system and can reduce pain intensity within minutes.

Progressive muscle relaxation can interrupt the pain-tension cycle. Starting with your toes, tense each muscle group for 5 seconds, then release. Work your way up your body, finishing with your face and scalp. This technique helps identify areas of tension you might not have noticed.

**Heat and Cold Applications**

Cold therapy works best for acute injuries, inflammation, and some types of headaches. Apply ice packs wrapped in a thin towel for 15-20 minutes, then remove for at least 20 minutes before reapplying. Never apply ice directly to skin, as this can cause frostbite.

Heat therapy is effective for muscle tension, chronic pain, and joint stiffness. Use heating pads, warm baths, or warm compresses for 15-20 minutes. Heat should be comfortably warm, not hot enough to burn. People with diabetes or circulation problems should use heat therapy cautiously.

Contrast therapy alternates between heat and cold applications. Start with heat for 3-4 minutes, then switch to cold for 1 minute. Repeat this cycle 3-4 times, ending with cold. This technique can be particularly effective for certain types of chronic pain.

**Positioning and Movement**

Proper positioning can significantly reduce pain intensity. For back pain, lie on your back with knees bent and feet flat on the floor, or lie on your side with a pillow between your knees. These positions reduce stress on the spine.

For neck pain, support your head with a rolled towel or small pillow, maintaining the natural curve of your neck. Avoid positions that force your head forward or backward.

Gentle movement often helps more than complete rest. Simple stretches, slow walking, or gentle range-of-motion exercises can prevent stiffness and reduce pain. Move within your comfort zone, stopping if pain worsens.

**Pressure Point Techniques**

The LI4 acupressure point, located in the webbing between your thumb and index finger, can help relieve headaches and general pain. Apply firm pressure for 1-2 minutes, then switch hands.

For headaches, apply pressure to the temples using circular motions. The GV20 point at the top of your head can also provide relief - apply gentle pressure for 30-60 seconds.

Foot reflexology points can address pain in various body parts. The area under your big toe corresponds to your head and neck, while the arch corresponds to your spine. Apply firm pressure to these areas for 1-2 minutes.

**Supplement Dosing Guidelines**

**Turmeric and Curcumin**

Standard curcumin dosing ranges from 500-1000mg taken twice daily with meals. Look for supplements that include piperine (black pepper extract) or are formulated as liposomal preparations for better absorption. Start with 500mg daily and increase gradually if needed.

Take curcumin with fat-containing meals to improve absorption. Avoid taking with iron supplements or blood-thinning medications without consulting your healthcare provider. Maximum recommended dose is 8-12 grams daily, though most people achieve benefits with much lower doses.

## Omega-3 Fatty Acids

For pain management, aim for 1-3 grams of combined EPA and DHA daily. Look for supplements that provide at least 1000mg of EPA, as this component appears most beneficial for pain relief. Take with meals to improve absorption and reduce stomach upset.

Fish oil supplements should be stored in the refrigerator and checked for freshness. Rancid fish oil can cause stomach upset and may not provide therapeutic benefits. Look for third-party tested products to ensure purity and potency.

## Magnesium

Magnesium glycinate or magnesium malate are generally better absorbed than magnesium oxide. Start with 200-400mg daily, taken with food to reduce stomach upset. The total daily dose can be divided between meals for better tolerance.

Magnesium can interact with certain medications, particularly antibiotics and heart medications. Take magnesium supplements at least 2 hours apart from these medications. Excessive magnesium can cause diarrhea, so reduce the dose if this occurs.

## Vitamin D

Most adults need 1000-4000 IU daily, depending on blood levels and sun exposure. Vitamin D3 is generally preferred over D2 for raising blood levels. Take with fat-containing meals for optimal absorption.

Blood testing helps determine your optimal dose. Levels should be maintained between 30-50 ng/mL for optimal health benefits. Some people may need higher doses, especially those with darker skin or limited sun exposure.

## Safety Considerations

Always consult healthcare providers before starting new supplements, especially if you take prescription medications. Many supplements can interact with medications or affect medical conditions.

Start with lower doses and increase gradually to assess tolerance. Keep a supplement log to track what you're taking and any effects you notice. Store supplements in cool, dry places away from direct sunlight.

## Red Flag Symptoms Requiring Immediate Care

### Neurological Warning Signs

Sudden, severe headache unlike any you've experienced before requires immediate medical attention. This could indicate a brain hemorrhage, stroke, or other serious condition. Associated symptoms like confusion, vision changes, or difficulty speaking make this an emergency.

New weakness or numbness in arms or legs, especially on one side of the body, suggests possible stroke or spinal cord injury. Don't wait to see if symptoms improve - seek immediate medical care.

Loss of bowel or bladder control with back pain could indicate cauda equina syndrome, a surgical emergency. This condition requires immediate treatment to prevent permanent nerve damage.

### Cardiovascular Symptoms

Chest pain, especially with shortness of breath, sweating, or nausea, requires immediate evaluation. These symptoms could indicate heart attack, even in people without known heart disease. Don't drive yourself to the hospital - call emergency services.

Sudden shortness of breath, especially with leg swelling or chest pain, could indicate pulmonary embolism. This life-threatening condition requires immediate medical attention.

### Infection Signs

Fever with severe pain, especially with redness, swelling, or warmth around the painful area, could indicate serious infection. Bone infections, abscesses, or blood infections require immediate treatment.

Neck stiffness with fever and headache suggests possible meningitis, a medical emergency. This combination of symptoms requires immediate hospital evaluation.

## Trauma-Related Concerns

Severe pain after head injury, especially with confusion, vomiting, or loss of consciousness, requires immediate medical evaluation. These symptoms could indicate serious brain injury.

Severe pain with obvious bone deformity, inability to move a limb, or loss of pulse or sensation suggests fracture or vascular injury requiring emergency care.

## Abdominal Emergencies

Severe abdominal pain with vomiting, especially if you can't keep fluids down, could indicate bowel obstruction or other surgical emergency. Sudden onset of severe abdominal pain requires immediate evaluation.

Severe pain with changes in bowel habits, blood in stool, or signs of dehydration needs prompt medical attention. These symptoms could indicate various serious conditions.

## Drug-Supplement Interactions

## Blood Thinning Interactions

Turmeric and curcumin can increase bleeding risk when combined with warfarin, aspirin, or other blood-thinning medications. The Cleveland Clinic recommends monitoring PT/INR levels more frequently if taking these combinations (110, 111, 112, 113).

Fish oil supplements can also increase bleeding risk, especially at doses above 3 grams daily. Inform your healthcare provider about all supplements before surgery or dental procedures.

Ginkgo biloba, garlic supplements, and high-dose vitamin E can also affect blood clotting. These interactions can be dangerous and require medical supervision.

### Diabetes Medication Interactions

Cinnamon supplements can lower blood sugar and may interact with diabetes medications. Monitor blood sugar levels more frequently if using cinnamon supplements with diabetes medications.

Chromium supplements can also affect blood sugar levels and may require diabetes medication adjustments. Work with your healthcare provider to monitor and adjust medications as needed.

### Blood Pressure Medication Interactions

Licorice root can increase blood pressure and reduce the effectiveness of blood pressure medications. Avoid licorice supplements if you have high blood pressure or take blood pressure medications.

Coenzyme Q10 may lower blood pressure and could interact with blood pressure medications. Monitor blood pressure regularly if taking this combination.

### Timing Considerations

Calcium and magnesium supplements can reduce absorption of certain antibiotics, particularly tetracyclines and fluoroquinolones. Take these supplements at least 2 hours apart from antibiotics.

Iron supplements can reduce absorption of several medications, including thyroid hormones and some antibiotics. Take iron supplements at least 2 hours apart from other medications.

Fiber supplements can affect absorption of many medications by binding to them in the digestive tract. Take fiber supplements at least 2 hours apart from medications to ensure proper absorption.

### Monitoring Requirements

Regular blood work may be needed when combining certain supplements with medications. Your healthcare provider can determine appropriate monitoring schedules based on your specific situation.

Keep detailed records of all supplements and medications you take, including dosages and timing. This information is crucial for healthcare providers to assess interaction risks.

Report any new symptoms or changes in existing symptoms to your healthcare provider, especially if they occur after starting new supplements or medications.

**Practical Application**

These quick reference guides provide immediate access to essential pain management information, but they don't replace professional medical care. Use these tools as part of your overall pain management strategy, not as substitutes for proper medical evaluation and treatment.

The emergency techniques can provide significant relief and help you manage pain crises more effectively. However, chronic pain requires ongoing professional management and shouldn't be handled solely through emergency measures.

Supplement dosing information provides starting points for discussions with healthcare providers. Individual needs vary based on health status, other medications, and specific conditions. Always consult with qualified healthcare professionals before making significant changes to your supplement regimen.

**Reference Resource Excellence**

These quick reference guides transform complex medical information into actionable tools you can use during pain crises. They provide the essential knowledge needed to manage pain safely and effectively while recognizing when professional help is necessary.

The key to successful pain management lies in preparation. By familiarizing yourself with these guides before you need them, you'll be better equipped to handle pain crises with confidence and appropriate action. Keep these resources easily accessible - in your phone, wallet, or posted in your home - so they're available when pain strikes.

**Quick Reference Essentials:**

- Emergency pain relief techniques provide immediate options for various pain types

- Evidence-based supplement dosing ensures safe and effective use

- Red flag symptoms help identify when immediate medical care is necessary

- Drug-supplement interactions prevent dangerous combinations

- Preparation and accessibility make these guides most effective during pain crises

- Professional medical care remains essential for chronic pain management

# Appendix B: Resources and Support

The journey through chronic pain can feel isolating, but you're not alone. Millions of people share similar experiences, and numerous organizations, professionals, and online communities exist to provide support, education, and advocacy. This appendix connects you with vetted resources that can enhance your pain management journey and provide ongoing support.

Finding quality resources requires discernment. The internet contains vast amounts of information about pain management, but not all sources are reliable or evidence-based. The resources listed here have been selected for their credibility, usefulness, and commitment to evidence-based information.

**Professional Organizations**

**American Chronic Pain Association (ACPA)**

The ACPA provides education, support, and advocacy for people with chronic pain conditions. Their website offers extensive educational materials, support group locators, and resources for families and caregivers. The organization focuses on helping people develop self-management skills and cope with chronic pain.

The ACPA offers peer support programs that connect people with chronic pain to others who understand their experiences. These programs provide emotional support and practical advice from people who have successfully managed their own chronic pain conditions.

**International Association for the Study of Pain (IASP)**

The IASP is the leading professional organization for pain researchers and clinicians worldwide. Their website provides current research findings, position statements, and educational resources. The Global Year Against Pain campaigns focus on specific pain conditions and provide comprehensive educational materials.

The IASP maintains professional standards for pain management and provides continuing education for healthcare providers. Their resources help ensure that pain management practices are based on current scientific evidence.

## American Pain Society (APS)

Although the APS dissolved in 2019, many of their educational resources remain available through other organizations. Their legacy includes evidence-based guidelines and educational materials that continue to influence pain management practices.

The dissolution of the APS highlighted the need for new organizations to fill the gap in pain education and advocacy. Several newer organizations have emerged to continue this important work.

## Specialized Condition Organizations

The Arthritis Foundation provides resources specifically for people with arthritis and related conditions. Their website offers exercise programs, educational materials, and support group locators. They also advocate for arthritis research and improved access to care.

The American Migraine Foundation focuses on headache and migraine education. Their resources include information about latest treatments, lifestyle modifications, and finding qualified healthcare providers.

The National Fibromyalgia and Chronic Pain Association provides resources for people with fibromyalgia and other chronic pain conditions. They offer educational materials, support groups, and advocacy efforts.

## Online Communities and Support Groups

## Vetted Support Communities

PainScale is a comprehensive online platform that combines pain tracking tools with community support. Users can track their pain patterns, connect with others who have similar conditions, and access educational resources. The platform is moderated to ensure quality discussions and prevent misinformation.

The Mighty is a social network for people with chronic conditions, including various pain conditions. The platform allows users to share experiences, ask questions, and find support from others who understand their challenges. Content is moderated to maintain a supportive environment.

### Condition-Specific Communities

CreakyJoints serves people with arthritis and related conditions. The platform provides educational content, advocacy opportunities, and community support. Users can connect with others who have similar diagnoses and share experiences about treatments and management strategies.

MyMigraineTriggers is a community focused on headache and migraine management. Users can track triggers, share experiences, and access educational content about migraine management. The platform emphasizes evidence-based information and practical management strategies.

### Safety in Online Communities

When joining online communities, protect your privacy by using screen names rather than real names. Be cautious about sharing personal medical information or contact details with other users.

Verify medical information with qualified healthcare providers before acting on advice from online communities. While peer support is valuable, it shouldn't replace professional medical guidance.

Report inappropriate behavior or misinformation to community moderators. Quality communities have systems in place to maintain supportive, accurate environments.

### Recommended Apps and Digital Tools

### Pain Tracking Applications

PainScale offers comprehensive pain tracking with weather correlation, medication tracking, and symptom monitoring. The app includes educational content and allows users to generate reports for healthcare providers.

ArthritisPower is developed by CreakyJoints and provides specialized tracking for arthritis symptoms. The app includes features for tracking joint pain, stiffness, and medication effectiveness.

Migraine Buddy specializes in headache and migraine tracking. The app helps users identify triggers, track medication effectiveness, and monitor patterns. It includes weather tracking and can generate reports for healthcare providers.

## Meditation and Relaxation Apps

Headspace offers guided meditations specifically designed for pain management. The app includes programs for chronic pain, stress reduction, and sleep improvement. Content is developed by qualified meditation teachers and healthcare professionals.

Calm provides sleep stories, meditation programs, and relaxation techniques. The app includes content specifically designed for pain management and stress reduction.

Insight Timer offers a large library of free meditations, including content specifically for pain management. The app includes programs by qualified teachers and healthcare professionals.

## Exercise and Movement Apps

Yoga for Chronic Pain provides gentle yoga routines designed specifically for people with chronic pain conditions. The app includes modifications for various limitations and emphasizes safety.

Pool Exercise App offers water-based exercise routines that are gentle on joints while providing effective movement therapy. The app includes programs for various pain conditions and fitness levels.

## Medication and Supplement Tracking

Medisafe provides medication reminders and tracking features. The app can help ensure consistent medication timing and provide records for healthcare providers.

MyRA tracks medications, symptoms, and appointments specifically for people with rheumatoid arthritis. The app can generate reports for healthcare providers and helps monitor treatment effectiveness.

## Educational Resources and Further Reading

### Evidence-Based Websites

The National Institute of Neurological Disorders and Stroke (NINDS) provides comprehensive information about pain, neurological conditions, and current research. Their resources are based on current scientific evidence and regularly updated.

The National Center for Complementary and Integrative Health (NCCIH) offers evidence-based information about complementary approaches to pain management. Their resources help people make informed decisions about alternative treatments.

### Professional Medical Websites

Mayo Clinic's website provides comprehensive information about pain conditions, treatments, and management strategies. Content is reviewed by medical professionals and based on current evidence.

Cleveland Clinic offers extensive resources about pain management, including information about various conditions and treatment approaches. Their content is regularly updated and medically reviewed.

### Books for Deeper Learning

"The Pain Chronicles" by Melanie Thernstrom provides a comprehensive look at pain from historical, scientific, and personal perspectives. The book offers insights into how pain affects individuals and society.

"Painful Yarns" by Lorimer Moseley uses storytelling to explain complex pain science concepts in accessible language. The book helps readers understand how pain works and how it can be managed.

"The Mindful Body" by Ellen Langer explores the connection between mind and body in health and healing. The book provides scientific insights into how thoughts and attitudes affect physical experiences.

## Research and Scientific Literature

PubMed provides access to medical research publications. While technical, this database allows readers to access the latest research findings about pain management and treatment approaches.

Cochrane Reviews offer systematic reviews of medical treatments, including pain management interventions. These reviews provide evidence-based assessments of treatment effectiveness.

## Advocacy and Policy Resources

## Patient Advocacy Organizations

The Alliance for the Treatment of Intractable Pain advocates for appropriate pain treatment and patient rights. The organization works to influence policy and improve access to effective pain management.

Pain Action focuses on advocacy and policy change to improve pain care. They work to influence healthcare policy and fight stigma associated with chronic pain conditions.

## Healthcare Policy Information

The American Medical Association provides information about healthcare policy changes that affect pain management. Their resources help patients understand how policy changes might impact their care.

The Centers for Disease Control and Prevention offers information about pain management guidelines and public health initiatives.

Their resources help patients understand evidence-based approaches to pain management.

## Building Your Support Network

### Combining Resources Effectively

Use multiple resources to create a comprehensive support network. Professional organizations provide credible information, online communities offer peer support, and apps help with practical management tasks.

Verify information across multiple sources before making treatment decisions. Cross-referencing information helps ensure accuracy and completeness.

### Maintaining Privacy and Safety

Protect your personal information when using online resources. Use strong passwords, enable two-factor authentication when available, and be cautious about sharing personal details.

Report scams or inappropriate behavior to platform administrators. Quality platforms have systems in place to maintain safe, supportive environments.

### Support Network Excellence

Building a strong support network requires time and effort, but the benefits are substantial. Quality resources provide education, emotional support, and practical tools that can significantly improve your pain management outcomes.

The key to successful resource utilization lies in selecting credible sources and using them appropriately. Professional organizations provide evidence-based information, online communities offer peer support, and apps help with practical management tasks. Used together, these resources create a comprehensive support system that can sustain you through your pain management journey.

**Resource and Support Strategies:**

- Professional organizations provide credible, evidence-based information and advocacy

- Online communities offer peer support and shared experiences from others with similar conditions

- Apps and digital tools help with practical management tasks like pain tracking and medication reminders

- Educational resources support informed decision-making about treatment options

- Advocacy organizations work to improve pain care and patient rights

- Building a comprehensive support network requires selecting credible sources and using them appropriately

# Appendix C: Worksheets and Tools

Effective pain management requires systematic tracking, clear goal-setting, and organized communication with healthcare providers. These worksheets and tools transform abstract concepts into practical applications you can use immediately. Think of them as your personal pain management laboratory - places to experiment, track, and refine your approach to managing chronic pain.

The tools in this appendix have been designed for real-world use, recognizing that pain can affect concentration and motivation. Each worksheet focuses on essential information while remaining simple enough to use even during difficult days. They provide structure for your pain management journey while allowing flexibility for your unique needs and circumstances.

## Pain Assessment and Tracking Forms

### Daily Pain Log

Date: _____

### Morning Assessment (upon waking)

- Pain intensity (0-10 scale): _____

- Primary pain location: _____

- Pain quality (circle all that apply): Burning, Aching, Stabbing, Throbbing, Cramping, Sharp, Dull, Other: _____

- Stiffness level (0-10): _____

- Sleep quality (1-5, 5 being excellent): _____

### Midday Assessment

- Pain intensity (0-10 scale): _____

- Any changes in pain location: _____

- Activity level this morning: _____

- Medications taken: _____

- Non-medication treatments used: _____

## Evening Assessment

- Pain intensity (0-10 scale): _____

- Overall function today (1-5, 5 being excellent): _____

- Stress level (0-10): _____

- Mood (circle one): Good, Fair, Poor, Anxious, Depressed, Irritable

- Activities completed today: _____

- Activities avoided due to pain: _____

## Weekly Review Questions

- What patterns do you notice in your pain levels?

- Which treatments were most helpful this week?

- What activities worsened your pain?

- What factors seemed to improve your pain?

- Any new symptoms or changes to report?

## Monthly Pain Assessment

## Overall Pain Patterns

- Average pain intensity this month: _____

- Number of "good" days (pain 0-3): _____

- Number of "moderate" days (pain 4-6): _____

- Number of "severe" days (pain 7-10): _____

**Functional Impact Assessment** Rate how pain affected each area this month (0 = no impact, 10 = completely unable to function):

- Work/school: _____

- Household activities: _____

- Social activities: _____

- Exercise/physical activity: _____

- Sleep: _____

- Mood: _____

- Relationships: _____

**Treatment Effectiveness Review** For each treatment you used this month, rate its effectiveness (1-5, 5 being very effective):

- Medication 1: _____ Rating: _____

- Medication 2: _____ Rating: _____

- Physical therapy: _____ Rating: _____

- Exercise: _____ Rating: _____

- Stress management: _____ Rating: _____

- Heat/cold therapy: _____ Rating: _____

- Other: _____ Rating: _____

**Trigger Identification** List factors that seemed to worsen your pain this month:

1. _____

2. _____

3. _____

List factors that seemed to improve your pain this month:

1. _____

2. _____

3. _____

## Goal-Setting Templates

## SMART Goals for Pain Management

**Goal #1:** Specific: What exactly do you want to achieve?

_____

Measurable: How will you measure progress?

_____

Achievable: Is this realistic given your current condition?

_____

Relevant: Why is this goal important to you?

_____

Time-bound: When do you want to achieve this goal?

_____

## Action Steps:

1. _____
2. _____
3. _____

## Potential Obstacles:

1. _____
2. _____

## Strategies to Overcome Obstacles:

1. _____
2. _____

## Support Needed:

246

**Progress Tracking Method:**

**3-Month Goal Planning Template**

**Physical Goals**

- Exercise goal: _____
- Activity goal: _____
- Sleep goal: _____

**Functional Goals**

- Work/school goal: _____
- Social goal: _____
- Self-care goal: _____

**Treatment Goals**

- Medication goal: _____
- Therapy goal: _____
- Self-management goal:

  _____

**Quality of Life Goals**

- Mood goal: _____
- Relationship goal: _____
- Hobby/interest goal: _____

**Medication and Supplement Tracking**

**Medication Log**

**Prescription Medications** Medication Name: _____

Dose: _____ Frequency: _____ Prescribing Doctor:

_____ Start Date: _____ Purpose:

_____ Side Effects Experienced:

_____ Effectiveness Rating (1-5):

_____

Medication Name: _____ Dose: _____ Frequency:

_____ Prescribing Doctor: _____ Start Date: _____

Purpose: _____ Side Effects

Experienced: _____ Effectiveness

Rating (1-5): _____

**Over-the-Counter Medications** Medication Name:

_____ Dose: _____ Frequency: _____ Purpose:

_____ Effectiveness Rating (1-5):

_____

**Supplements** Supplement Name: _____ Dose: _____

Frequency: _____ Brand: _____ Start Date: _____

Purpose: _____ Effectiveness

Rating (1-5): _____

**Medication Timing Log** Create a weekly grid showing when you take
each medication:

Monday: _____ Tuesday:

_____ Wednesday:

_____ Thursday:

_____ Friday:

_____ Saturday:

_____ Sunday:

_____

**Side Effect Tracking** Date: _____ Medication: _____

Side Effect: _____ Severity (1-5): _____ Duration:

_____ Action Taken: _____

**Pharmacy and Refill Information** Pharmacy Name:

_____ Phone: _____ Pharmacy

Address: _____ Preferred
Pharmacist: _____

**Medication Refill Schedule** Medication: _____ Last
Refill: _____ Next Refill Due: _____ Medication:
_____ Last Refill: _____ Next Refill Due: _____

## Healthcare Provider Communication Tools

## Pre-Appointment Preparation

**Appointment Date:** _____ **Provider:** _____ **Time:**

_____

## Primary Concerns to Discuss:

1. _____

2. _____

3. _____

## Questions to Ask:

1. _____

2. _____

3. _____

## Symptoms to Report:

- New symptoms since last visit: _____

- Changes in existing symptoms: _____

- Side effects from medications: _____

## Current Treatment Effectiveness:

- What's working well: _____

- What's not working: _____

- Changes you'd like to make: _____

**Appointment Notes Template**

Date: _____ Provider: _____ Duration: _____

**Provider's Assessment:**

_____

**Recommendations:**

   1. _____

   2. _____

   3. _____

**New Prescriptions or Changes:**

_____

**Tests or Referrals Ordered:**

_____

**Follow-up Instructions:**

_____

**Next Appointment:** Date: _____ Time: _____ Purpose:

_____

**Questions for Healthcare Providers**

**About Your Condition:**

- What is causing my pain?

- How might my condition change over time?

- What are my treatment options?

- What are the benefits and risks of each option?

- How will we know if treatments are working?

**About Medications:**

- How does this medication work?

- What side effects should I watch for?

- How long before I see improvement?

- What should I do if I miss a dose?

- Can this medication interact with my other medications?

**About Lifestyle Management:**

- What activities should I avoid?

- What exercises are safe for me?

- How can I manage stress effectively?

- What dietary changes might help?

- How can I improve my sleep?

**About Resources:**

- What support groups do you recommend?

- Are there educational resources specific to my condition?

- What specialists might be helpful?

- How can I stay informed about new treatments?

**Treatment Planning Worksheet**

**Current Treatment Plan Review**

**What's Working Well:**

1. _____

2. _____

3. _____

**What's Not Working:**

1. _____

2. _____

3. _____

**What's Missing:**

1. _____

2. _____

3. _____

**New Approaches to Try:**

1. _____

2. _____

3. _____

**Barriers to Treatment:**

1. _____

2. _____

3. _____

**Resources Needed:**

1. _____

2. _____

3. _____

**Personal Pain Management Reference**

**Emergency Contacts:** Primary Care Doctor: _____
Phone: _____ Pain Specialist: _____
Phone: _____ Pharmacy: _____ Phone:
_____ Emergency Contact: _____
Phone: _____

**Medical Information:** Blood Type: _____ Allergies:
_____ Current Medications:
_____ Medical Conditions:
_____ Insurance Information:
_____

**Personal Pain Management Kit:**

- Medications currently taking:

  _____

- Comfort items that help:

  _____

- Relaxation techniques that work:

  _____

- Activities that worsen pain:

  _____

- Activities that improve pain:

  _____

**Practical Implementation**

These worksheets and tools work best when used consistently over time. Start with one or two tools that seem most relevant to your current needs, then gradually add others as you become comfortable with the process.

The key to success is finding the right balance between thoroughness and practicality. You want enough information to identify patterns and guide treatment decisions, but not so much detail that tracking becomes burdensome.

Consider using digital versions of these tools if you prefer technology-based tracking. Many smartphone apps can replicate these functions while providing additional features like reminders and data analysis.

**Tool Mastery**

These worksheets and tools transform pain management from a vague process into a systematic approach. They provide structure for tracking your progress, setting realistic goals, and communicating effectively with healthcare providers.

The power of these tools lies not in their complexity but in their consistent use. By regularly tracking your pain patterns, setting clear goals, and preparing for healthcare appointments, you become an active participant in your pain management rather than a passive recipient of care.

**Worksheet and Tool Essentials:**

- Pain assessment forms provide systematic tracking of symptoms, triggers, and treatment effectiveness

- Goal-setting templates help create realistic, measurable objectives for improvement

- Medication logs ensure safe, organized management of complex treatment regimens

- Healthcare provider communication tools improve the quality and efficiency of medical appointments

- Treatment planning worksheets help evaluate and adjust your pain management approach

- Consistent use of these tools transforms pain management from reactive to proactive

**Closing Reflection**

The journey through chronic pain is deeply personal, yet it follows patterns that can be understood, predicted, and modified. This book has provided you with evidence-based tools, practical strategies, and the knowledge needed to transform your relationship with pain from one of helplessness to one of empowerment.

The most important lesson is that effective pain management isn't about eliminating all discomfort - it's about reducing pain to manageable levels while maximizing your ability to live a meaningful, fulfilling life. The approaches outlined in these pages have helped millions of people achieve this goal, and they can help you too.

Your pain experience is unique, and your path to relief will be equally individual. Use the information in this book as a starting point, but don't hesitate to adapt, modify, and personalize these approaches to fit your specific needs and circumstances. The best pain management plan is the one you'll actually follow consistently.

The future of pain management is bright, with new treatments, technologies, and understanding emerging regularly. By staying informed, maintaining hope, and actively participating in your care, you position yourself to benefit from these advances while building the skills needed for long-term success.

Pain may have brought you to this book, but knowledge, tools, and determination will carry you forward. The journey continues, but now you have the resources to navigate it with confidence and hope.

# References

(1) Centers for Disease Control and Prevention. Wide-ranging online data for epidemiologic research (WONDER). Atlanta, GA: CDC, National Center for Health Statistics; 2020.

(2) Qaseem A, Wilt TJ, McLean RM, et al. Noninvasive treatments for acute, subacute, and chronic low back pain: a clinical practice guideline from the American College of Physicians. Ann Intern Med. 2017;166(7):514-530.

(3) Dowell D, Ragan KR, Jones CM, et al. CDC clinical practice guideline for prescribing opioids for pain — United States, 2022. MMWR Recomm Rep. 2022;71(3):1-95.

(4) Vertex Pharmaceuticals. FDA approves JOURNAVX™ (suzetrigine) for the management of moderate to severe acute pain in adults. Press release. January 2025.

(5) Zakrzewska JM, Palmer J, Morisset V, et al. Safety and efficacy of a Nav1.7 selective sodium channel blocker in patients with trigeminal neuralgia: a double-blind, placebo-controlled, randomised withdrawal phase 2a trial. Lancet Neurol. 2017;16(4):291-300.

(6) Gatchel RJ, McGeary DD, McGeary CA, et al. Interdisciplinary chronic pain management: past, present, and future. Am Psychol. 2014;69(2):119-130.

(7) American Pain Society. Interdisciplinary pain management. Glenview, IL: American Pain Society; 2010.

(8) Melzack R, Wall PD. Pain mechanisms: a new theory. Science. 1965;150(3699):971-979.

(9) Apkarian AV, Bushnell MC, Treede RD, et al. Human brain mechanisms of pain perception and regulation in health and disease. Eur J Pain. 2005;9(4):463-484.

(10) May A. Chronic pain may change the structure of the brain. Pain. 2008;137(1):7-15.

(11) Centers for Disease Control and Prevention. Chronic pain and high-impact chronic pain in U.S. adults, 2023. NCHS Data Brief. 2024;518:1-8.

(12) Gaskin DJ, Richard P. The economic costs of pain in the United States. J Pain. 2012;13(8):715-724.

(13) Centers for Disease Control and Prevention. Understanding the opioid overdose epidemic. Atlanta, GA: CDC; 2022.

(14) Journal of International Crisis and Risk Communication Research. Effectiveness of Physical Therapy for Chronic Pain Management. 2024.

(15) National Center for Complementary and Integrative Health. Chronic Pain and Complementary Health Approaches: Usefulness and Safety. 2024.

(16) UCLA Health. 5 alternative treatments for chronic pain. 2024.

(17) American College of Physicians. Noninvasive treatments for acute, subacute, and chronic low back pain: a clinical practice guideline. 2017.

(18) American College of Physicians. Acupuncture for chronic pain: individual patient data meta-analysis. 2012.

(19) American College of Physicians. Clinical practice guidelines for chronic pain management. 2017.

(20) American College of Physicians. Massage therapy for chronic pain conditions. 2017.

(21) Cochrane Database of Systematic Reviews. Spinal manipulative therapy for chronic low-back pain. 2019.

(22) Centers for Disease Control and Prevention. Nonopioid therapies for pain management. 2022.

(23) BioMed Central. Efficacy of virtual reality for pain relief in medical procedures: a systematic review and meta-analysis. 2024.

(24) PubMed Central. Virtual reality and pain management: current trends and future directions. 2023.

(25) PubMed Central. Spinal cord stimulation for chronic pain: a systematic review. 2023.

(26) PubMed Central. Peripheral nerve stimulation for chronic pain management. 2023.

(27) PubMed Central. Transcranial magnetic stimulation for chronic pain conditions. 2023.

(28) PubMed Central. Neuromodulation devices for pain management: current evidence. 2024.

(29) American College of Physicians. Heat therapy for acute and chronic pain conditions. 2017.

(30) American College of Physicians. Cold therapy applications in pain management. 2017.

(31) Cleveland Clinic Journal of Medicine. Central sensitization, chronic pain, and other symptoms: Better understanding, better management. 2023.

(32) Wikipedia. Mindfulness-based stress reduction. 2024.

(33) PubMed Central. Mindfulness-based stress reduction: a non-pharmacological approach for chronic illnesses. 2012.

(34) American College of Physicians. Mindfulness-based interventions for chronic pain management. 2017.

(35) Cleveland Clinic Journal of Medicine. Mindfulness-based stress reduction for chronic pain. 2023.

(36) PubMed Central. Hypnotherapy for the Management of Chronic Pain. 2009.

(37) ScienceDirect. Hypnosis to manage musculoskeletal and neuropathic chronic pain: A systematic review and meta-analysis. 2022.

(38) PubMed Central. Hypnotic Approaches for Chronic Pain Management: Clinical Implications of Recent Research Findings. 2015.

(39) Annals of Palliative Medicine. The role of clinical hypnosis and self-hypnosis to relief pain and anxiety in severe chronic diseases in palliative care. 2018.

(40) PubMed Central. Neurophysiology of pain and hypnosis for chronic pain. 2013.

(41) PubMed Central. Use of Hypnosis in the Treatment of Pain. 2012.

(42) Arthritis Foundation. Hypnosis for Pain Relief. 2024.

(43) ScienceDirect. The effectiveness of hypnosis for pain relief: A systematic review and meta-analysis. 2018.

(44) Stanford Medicine. How hypnosis can alter the brain's perception of pain. 2023.

(45) WebMD. Alternative Treatments for Chronic Pain: Hypnosis. 2024.

(46) Cleveland Clinic. Biofeedback: What It Is, Purpose, Procedure, Risks & Benefits. 2024.

(47) WebMD. Biofeedback Therapy: Uses and Benefits. 2024.

(48) PubMed Central. The Effect of Diaphragmatic Breathing on Attention, Negative Affect and Stress in Healthy Adults. 2017.

(49) PubMed Central. Effects of Diaphragmatic Breathing on Health: A Narrative Review. 2020.

(50) PubMed Central. Effectiveness of diaphragmatic breathing for reducing physiological and psychological stress in adults. 2019.

(51) Cleveland Clinic. Diaphragmatic Breathing Exercises & Benefits. 2024.

(52) VA. Diaphragmatic Breathing to Assist with Self-Management of Pain. 2024.

(53) University of Michigan Health. Diaphragmatic Breathing for GI Patients. 2024.

(54) PubMed Central. Diaphragmatic breathing exercises in recovery from fatigue-induced changes in spinal mobility. 2023.

(55) PubMed Central. Mindfulness meditation—based pain relief: a mechanistic account. 2016.

(56) Arthritis Foundation. Anti-Inflammatory Diet Do's and Don'ts. 2024.

(57) Harvard Health. Foods that fight inflammation. 2024.

(58) PubMed Central. Mediterranean Diet as a Tool to Combat Inflammation and Chronic Diseases. 2020.

(59) WebMD. Turmeric and Curcumin: Health, Spice, and Supplement Information. 2024.

(60) Johns Hopkins Medicine. Turmeric Benefits. 2024.

(61) Healthline. 10 Health Benefits of Turmeric and Curcumin. 2024.

(62) Harvard Health. Do glucosamine and chondroitin supplements actually work for arthritis? 2024.

(63) Arthritis Foundation. Glucosamine, Chondroitin for Osteoarthritis Pain. 2024.

(64) NCCIH. Glucosamine and Chondroitin for Osteoarthritis. 2024.

(65) PubMed Central. Effectiveness and safety of glucosamine and chondroitin for osteoarthritis. 2018.

(66) Mayo Clinic. Glucosamine. 2024.

(67) Cleveland Clinic. Glucosamine Chondroitin Supplement: Uses & Side Effects. 2024.

(68) WebMD. Glucosamine: Overview, Uses, Side Effects, Precautions. 2024.

(69) ScienceDirect. Efficacy and safety of glucosamine sulfate in osteoarthritis management. 2024.

(70) New England Journal of Medicine. Glucosamine, Chondroitin Sulfate, and the Two in Combination for Painful Knee Osteoarthritis. 2006.

(71) Healthline. Glucosamine Chondroitin: Uses, Benefits, Side Effects, and Dosage. 2024.

(72) American College of Physicians. Noninvasive treatments for acute, subacute, and chronic low back pain: a clinical practice guideline. 2017.

(73) American College of Physicians. Clinical practice guidelines for low back pain management. 2017.

(74) American College of Physicians. Evidence-based treatments for back pain. 2017.

(75) American College of Physicians. Physical therapy for low back pain. 2017.

(76) American College of Physicians. Manual therapy for spinal conditions. 2017.

(77) American College of Rheumatology. 2019 ACR/Arthritis Foundation Guideline for the Management of Osteoarthritis. 2019.

(78) NCCIH. Chronic Pain and Complementary Health Approaches: Usefulness and Safety. 2024.

(79) American Academy of Family Physicians. Fibromyalgia: Diagnosis and Management. 2023.

(80) American Academy of Family Physicians. Comprehensive fibromyalgia management. 2023.

(81) American Academy of Family Physicians. Evidence-based fibromyalgia treatment. 2023.

(82) PR Newswire. American Headache Society Publishes Updated Guidance on Migraine Preventive Therapy. 2024.

(83) Medscape. Migraine Headache Guidelines: Guidelines Summary. 2024.

(84) PubMed. Management of Adults With Acute Migraine: Evidence Assessment. 2024.

(85) NCBI. Pain Management Medications - StatPearls. 2024.

(86) NCBI. Gabapentin: Uses, Side Effects, Dosages, Interactions. 2024.

(87) NCBI. Nutritional Supplement for Neuropathic Pain Management. 2024.

(88) NCBI. Pharmacological management of neuropathic pain. 2024.

(89) NCBI. Diabetic neuropathy treatment approaches. 2024.

(90) ScienceDirect. Alternative therapies in chronic non-cancer pain management: A scoping review. 2025.

(91) International Association for the Study of Pain. What Do We Mean By Integrative Pain Care? 2024.

(92) International Association for the Study of Pain. Evidence-based integrative pain medicine. 2024.

(93) International Association for the Study of Pain. Integrative Medicine Approaches for Pain Management. 2024.

(94) International Association for the Study of Pain. Integrative Medicine for Pain Management in Oncology. 2024.

(95) International Association for the Study of Pain. Using Integrative Medicine in Pain Management. 2024.

(96) International Association for the Study of Pain. Multimodal, integrative therapies for pain management. 2024.

(97) International Association for the Study of Pain. Integrative Pain Medicine: The Science and Practice. 2024.

(98) International Association for the Study of Pain. Chronic Pain and Complementary Health Approaches. 2024.

(99) International Association for the Study of Pain. Academic pain medicine research approaches. 2024.

(100) Oxford Academic. Patient–Provider Interactions in the Management of Chronic Pain. 2024.

(101) Psychology Today. Pain Provider Red Flags. 2024.

(102) NCBI. Postoperative Pain Control - StatPearls. 2024.

(103) NCBI. Multimodal analgesia approaches for surgical pain. 2024.

(104) Surgery. Multimodal analgesia and alternatives to opioids for postoperative analgesia. 2024.

(105) PLOS. The effectiveness of physiotherapy interventions on pain and quality of life in adults with persistent post-surgical pain. 2024.

(106) UCLA Health. Elderly pain management strategies. 2024.

(107) Cleveland Clinic. Pregnancy and pain management safety guidelines. 2024.

(108) Labiotech. New non-opioid pain medication: What is in the pipeline in 2025? 2024.

(109) Labiotech. LTG compound development for acute pain treatment. 2024.

(110) Cleveland Clinic. Turmeric - Ibuprofen Interaction Details. 2024.

(111) Cleveland Clinic. Gabapentin: Uses, Side Effects, Dosages, Interactions. 2024.

(112) Cleveland Clinic. Supplement-drug interactions in pain management. 2024.

(113) Cleveland Clinic. Safe supplement use with chronic pain medications. 2024.

www.ingramcontent.com/pod-product-compliance
Lightning Source LLC
Chambersburg PA
CBHW062206270326
41930CB00009B/1664